A Good Life

A Good Life

The Power of Palliative Care

Jerry Pinto

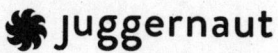

JUGGERNAUT BOOKS
C-I-128, First Floor, Sangam Vihar, Near Holi Chowk,
New Delhi 110080, India

First published by Juggernaut Books 2025

Copyright © Veha Foundation 2025

10 9 8 7 6 5 4 3 2 1

P-ISBN: 9789353459369
E-ISBN: 9789353458379

The views and opinions expressed in this book are the author's own. The facts contained herein were reported to be true as on the date of publication by the author to the publishers of the book, and the publishers are not in any way liable for their accuracy or veracity.

As is inevitable with a group of professionals who are in great demand, some of those interviewed here may have taken up new assignments. The designations and titles mentioned here are those that were current and correct at the time of writing.

All rights reserved. No part of this publication may be reproduced, transmitted, or stored in a retrieval system in any form or by any means without the written permission of the publisher.

Typeset in Adobe Caslon Pro by R. Ajith Kumar, Noida

Printed at Thomson Press India Ltd

Contents

Foreword by Rumana Hamied — ix

1. Ignorance Is Not Bliss — 1
2. Living Fully — 13
3. The Science and Art of Palliative Care — 35
4. An Interdisciplinary Approach to Healthcare — 55
5. Comfort, Where You Are — 93
6. Listening and Sharing — 119
7. Patient Navigators — 153
8. The Hidden Cost of Caring — 181
9. Integrating Palliative Care into Healthcare — 211
10. A Good Life — 237

Notes — 253
How Can I Find Palliative Care? — 255
Acknowledgements — 257

What Is Palliative Care

It is an inclusive approach to medical care for any serious illness, at any age, right from the moment of diagnosis. Care that helps you be as pain free as possible, allowing you to find joy and peace amidst your journey. Care that keeps you and your family at the heart. A true partnership between medical professionals and yourself, which accompanies you in your most difficult of times.

Foreword

Reading Jerry Pinto's seminal novel *Em and the Big Hoom* compelled me to seek him out.

Few voices capture the onerous, often unspoken burdens of life in prose as delicately and insightfully as Jerry's. His deeply personal narrative draws us into the everyday struggles of his family, bound by love and tested by the complexities of his mother's mental illness, revealing layers of vulnerability and endurance. His family navigated incredibly overwhelming challenges without holistic, supportive care, yet they miraculously managed to remain unshakably committed to each other. Their suffering was not inevitable, they should have been embraced with care. How were they not? Why were they not? For the last two decades, these questions have guided my personal search to bring this care within reach, so we don't fail others like Jerry.

When Jerry and I finally met, he told me what I had already divined from his book – that he had not known about palliative care. And that no one had needed it more than his mother; than him. His family was not offered an additional layer of support, mitigating suffering, easing symptoms, anchoring them in capable, compassionate care. We spoke about how this care might not have been as readily accessible back then, but it exists today, and with Jerry's voice, more people in need could find their way to it through greater awareness.

Now, two years later, I'm thrilled that with this book Jerry brings this to light through his insightful journey into palliative care. He has travelled across the length and breadth of India, meeting, engaging, learning and listening to people who are at the heart of this care – medical professionals, patients and families seeking to answer the most fundamental questions of what we deserve, what we need and what we get when we are seriously ill. While serving as a guide, this book lays out the unique landscape of palliative care in India, inviting all those facing serious illnesses to find the right care and comfort they need. It emphatically alerts us that palliative care should start at diagnosis, allowing both adults and children with serious illnesses to live fully and meaningfully.

My own understanding of palliative care began in 1993. I was just about twenty-one when my father took me to see a barren plot of land on the outskirts of Pune. It was there that I first heard the term 'palliative care'. He told me this land would hold a place where people with serious illnesses, along with their families, could find relief from pain and helplessness. 'It will be free, of course,' he said, 'because you can't be tranquil if you're worrying about doctors' bills.'

The Cipla Palliative Care and Training Centre opened in Warje, Pune, in 1997, built around a community courtyard, the *aangan*, with wards named after flowers to bring beauty into a medical setting. Here, patients are known by their names, not bed numbers – each one a story, a life. Loved ones are not left on the sidelines but are invited to stay, learning the art of caregiving while finding strength and solace themselves.

Five years later, I witnessed the gift of palliative care first-hand when my dearest friend Hazel D'Souza's cancer returned, in its final stages. We sat up with her, bracing ourselves as she cried out in pain. She had seen our centre in Pune and asked to be moved there. On her first night at the centre, with her pain finally managed, Hazel slept peacefully for eight hours straight – and so did we, after weeks of sleepless vigils. Hazel had only a few weeks left, and she spent them at the centre, free of pain. That, in the end, was what mattered most to all of us who loved her.

I will always remember a story my father shared about what palliative care means to him. 'For me, it's summed up by an incident about ten years after the centre opened,' he said. 'An elderly patient asked who I was. When he learned that I had helped to set up the place, he insisted on speaking with me. He said, "*Bhau* (brother), this is the place where I first understood the meaning of the word love." My father hugged him because in that simple statement lay the essence of palliative care.'

If we think of healthcare in terms of numbers alone, we miss the big picture of our country's health story. But if we think of stories like those of Hazel,

Foreword

the love-touched elderly gentleman, and thousands of others that Cipla's palliative care centre has served since it began, we can hope that access to palliative care for all can be possible – and perhaps even dream that light can be shone into the darkest corners.

In this book, you'll meet many incredible palliative care professionals, team members, volunteers and more, each guiding patients and families through illness. For palliative care is a collective effort where everyone plays a part – from the nurse to the ward boy, from the attendant to the counsellor. In each chapter, Jerry takes us into the lives of people facing illness, bringing us close to their courage, their humour, their sorrows and the resilience of those who care for them.

I hope these stories bring you alive to palliative care and deepen your understanding of the challenges of living with serious illnesses. Both you and I need it more than we know. Our parents already do. We are caregivers already and some of us will need caregivers sooner than we imagine. Who will stand with us then? Only a palliative care approach to medicine will be able to come through for us. And that care is possible, and every day people are seeking it out.

These are stories of hope and joy, pain and loss. Jerry's, mine, yours. Universal, binding, uncomplicated – we love, and we are loved. And we deserve to be able to give those we love a good life.

Rumana Hamied
Director
Veha Foundation

1
Ignorance Is Not Bliss

I wish I had known about palliative care earlier.

I wish my parents had known about it, too. After I was born in 1966, my mother began to experience depression. The doctors dismissed this as a post-partum phenomenon. It happens, they said, it will pass. Take up knitting, they said. Within six months, she had thrown herself in front of a bus. She survived. Passers-by put her into a taxi where she sat cross-legged and apologized again and again to the taxi driver for dirtying his car with the blood flowing from the wound on her foot.

In the hospital bed, she must have wondered what had gone wrong. She had not had it easy – a refugee from Burma, a child making a wartime crossing, an adolescent who wanted to be a teacher but who was forced to become a stenographer because companies paid better salaries than schools and money was needed at home. But she was no different in her troubles from thousands of other women, and they were not trying to kill themselves.

Up until then, my parents were a bright young couple on the ascent. They had a library that was the envy of their friends in Bombay. My mother wrote beautifully – her letters to my father, an engineer with blue eyes – an abiding delight. She sang for a while in the Paranjoti Choir of the city. She was known as a warm, witty woman with a job in the American consulate, which my father had found for her. They hung out in bookshops and loitered over Coke floats at Bombelli's. They married late and settled into a one BHK in Mahim. A year later, their first child, Andrea, was born. Then I came along, and something threw a switch in our mother's brain.

After her first suicide attempt, the doctors stopped telling her to count her blessings, to pull herself together and to think of those less fortunate than her. They said she was bipolar, and that there was no cure. She would have to learn to live with it. And with a prescription, they turned my parents out into the world to make the best of it. The doctors did not mean badly.

They did the best they could. They were not trained to think about suffering, nor even pain.

Dr M.R. Rajagopal, the founder of Pallium India, dedicated to increasing access to palliative care throughout the country, would have been a young medical student the year that my mother became ill. He was among the first people I met when I started writing this book. 'I had an excellent medical education,' he told me as we sipped coffee at his office in Thiruvananthapuram. 'We had the finest doctors teaching us. But never once did they mention pain or suffering. It was there. We knew it because we could hear the moans and the screams. But my generation of doctors were not taught to deal with it or even acknowledge it.' As I would discover through the course of writing this book, only now is this beginning to change in our country – or, indeed, in much of the world.

I have lost count of how many times my mother tried to end her life. She's gone now, and the nightmare has ended. Time has begun the sealing over of life's wounds, leaving only memories of her raucous laugh, her witty retorts, her self-mocking humour and her sharp sense of the ridiculous.

But when I heard of palliative care, something inside me started a low keening. It was the age-old song of 'What if'. What if my mother had had access to palliative care? What if there had been someone she could call when she was depressed and found it hard to breathe, when she did not want to breathe? What if she had someone to call and say, 'I want to die. I want them to kill me, but they won't'? What if I had had someone to call and say, 'She wants us to kill her and if she asks again, I'm worried I just might'?

My sister, the quiet one, capable of huge acts of empathy in her silence and by just being there, bore the brunt of it. What if she had had someone to offer her a hand? What if my sister and I had had a place where we could go to talk about our anger and our hurt – and the attendant guilt we felt when we prayed or wished or longed for a 'normal' mother? What if I had had someone to look me in the eye and say, 'This is not your fault'?

In *Em and the Big Hoom*, the novel that I wrote about life with our mother, Em, the manic-depressive superstar of her own drama, dies in her sleep, leaving her family shell-shocked and adrift. I wrote it like that because I knew that I had to open the door of the tiny Mahim flat in which the novel was set and let the readers out. I had to release the pressure. But that was not how it worked out in real life. There, my father died at fifty-nine, exhausted by carrying so many responsibilities, felled by his first and last heart attack. And that left the three of us to figure things out the best we could. We pulled through somehow, but it would have been so much easier on all of us if we had had someone to walk with us, someone with whom we could have talked about our pain.

Pain is an inevitable part of human life; it is an evolutionary gift, our best teacher. To be born without the ability to feel pain may sound like a blessing, but it is actually a terrible disability that hastens death because pain alerts us to a problem in the body that needs attention. Steps can then be taken, whether these are reflex actions or conscious steps, to alleviate the pain and to address the underlying problem. We need to accept then that pain is inevitable. But *suffering* need not be. Palliative care seeks to lessen both the pain and the suffering caused by illness.

I have since forgiven myself for the gaps in my knowledge of palliative care. When a medical stalwart like Dr Armida Fernandez, ex-dean of Lokmanya Tilak Municipal Medical College and General Hospital, Mumbai (otherwise known as Sion Hospital), neonatologist, and founder of Asia's first human milk bank, tells me that she had not heard of palliative care, how could I have possibly known? Early in the writing of this book, I met this redoubtable octogenarian who still visits daily the Romila Palliative Care Centre in Mumbai, which she founded. She told me about her family's brush with cancer.

Her daughter Romila was a precious child, born after many years of waiting. The infant had health issues: acute jaundice that meant her blood had to be completely changed, which could have caused other developmental delays. But she came through it all.

And then, at the age of sixteen or seventeen, 'Romila was diagnosed with Hodgkin lymphoma when it was already stage 3,' says Dr Armida.

Romila's education was to suffer a setback because her college would not accept her illness as a reason for poor attendance. Undeterred, she shifted to a women's university and finished her degree. Dr Armida tells me of Romila's love for life and her compassion for others. But then the cancer returned. 'Fourteen years later, she developed cancer of the breast. This may have been caused by the radiation she'd had for Hodgkin. Radiation itself can cause cancer,' says Dr Armida.

The young woman died, leaving behind a bereaved husband and a grieving family. 'When I lost Romila to cancer, there was pain and anguish. No one had heard of palliative care,' Dr Armida says. So when she did hear of palliative care, she decided that it was something she could do for others. She had already founded a community-driven NGO in Mumbai called SNEHA (Society for Nutrition, Education, and Health Action) to improve the health and well-being of vulnerable women and children. To its ambit, she added palliative care.

Beyond this, Dr Armida has now become an advocate of palliative care. 'I enjoyed teaching neonatology at Sion Hospital. Retiring as the head of the department means many generations of doctors have worked with me. Some of my students teach at neonatology colleges and all of them have been sensitized to the need for palliative care. I spread the message of palliative care wherever I go,' she adds.

As she tells me this, Dr Armida has no idea that Romila and she have managed another healing. Listening to her, I put down my guilt. We just did not know, Dr Armida and I. But we're trying to do something about it now. Dr Armida with her tireless advocacy, and I, by writing this book.

This book seeks to start a conversation about what palliative care is, challenges the misperceptions around it, and addresses who needs it and where it can be found. It is meant for all doctors who would like to shape a better life for their patients. It is meant for carers in the family who find their resources stretched but do not know that help could be a phone call away in some cities. It hopes to reassure everyone who is dealing with chronic illness or life-limiting conditions that there is no shame in asking for help. In fact, the shame should be ours as a society if there is no help to hand.

You cannot undo the past. But you can remake the present. By what we know, by what you will know at the end of reading this book, we will effect change. We will talk about palliative care to each other. We will be the change we want to see.

2
Living Fully

Dr Mary Ann Muckaden, who started the Palliative Care Unit at Tata Memorial Hospital (TMH),[1] Mumbai, in 1996, explains palliative care very simply: 'It focuses on living, not dying. It's a holistic approach that supports patients and their families physically, emotionally, socially and spiritually, starting from diagnosis. It's not about choosing between quality and quantity of life – palliative care can help you have both by helping you live as well as you can, for as long as you can.'

More formally, the World Health Organization (WHO) defines palliative care as 'an approach that improves the quality of life of patients (adults and children) and their families facing problems associated with life-threatening illness. It prevents and relieves suffering through the early identification, correct assessment, and treatment of pain and other problems, whether physical, psychosocial or spiritual.'[2]

Most of the key players in India's burgeoning palliative care movement have used this definition as a springboard rather than a straitjacket. They have expanded the understanding of a life-threatening illness to take in conditions that also limit how fully someone can live. This can include old age, for a nonagenarian who falls and fractures a rib and finds even taking a breath painful may need pain relief and emotional support as much as a cancer patient. It also extends to any chronic complex illness such as cardiac problems, neurological disorders like dementia and Parkinson's, as well as conditions like thalassemia.

While we stand in awe of the improvements in medicine, it would surprise most people to know how many diseases can, in reality, be cured. The National Library of Medicine (NLM) reckons that there are 26,000 diseases representing all areas of the body. Some of these are curable, many are not.

Dr Nandini Vallath, head of the Department of Pain and Palliative Medicine at St John's Medical College Hospital, Bengaluru, tells me, 'When I talk to a batch of young doctors, I ask them: What do you think will be the percentage of the diseases that you will see during your career that you can cure? The answer is generally anything between 60 and 70 per cent. The truth is closer to 10 to 15 per cent. There are a few infections, some nutritional issues, some minor and moderate tumours, and some mild to moderate traumas that we can cure. The rest will become chronic conditions. We can manage them, we can control or retard them, but they will advance. They will persist for a lifetime, they will change the way one interacts with one's body, they will rewrite one's relationship with the world. And there will come a point when we must ask ourselves: "Is what I am prescribing harming more than it is helping?"'

Dr Mamta Manglani, director, Academic and Research at the Comprehensive Thalassemia Care PBCF-MCGM, Mumbai, says, 'Medicine traditionally focused on diagnosing and curing illnesses, trying to restore health and treat the disease. But for people with chronic or life-limiting conditions, a cure isn't always possible. That's where palliative care comes in. It focuses on improving quality of life by managing pain, easing emotional distress and supporting both patients and their families. I've seen how powerful palliative care can be in managing symptoms and guiding families through tough decisions. And this matters just as much as the medical treatments themselves.'

Think of a child with severe juvenile diabetes who must not eat cake at a party or pop the sweet offered in class when it is someone's birthday into their mouth. Think of a young man diagnosed with amyotrophic lateral sclerosis (ALS), whose nerve cells, spinal cord and brain are degenerating to the extent that he will soon be unable to walk without support, and how this will affect his work life and his personal life, a life that is going to be cut short painfully and dramatically. Think of a senior citizen who can no longer tie their shoelaces or drink their soup because of Parkinson's disease. Think of how difficult it would be to battle this alone, to have to depend only on the family and the demands it places on our loved ones.

So if doctors can only cure 10 to 15 per cent of what ails humanity, surely they should be willing to expand their remit from curing the patient to caring for the patient? 'Unfortunately,' says Dr Vallath, 'these are not questions raised in mainstream clinical training and practice.'

To appreciate palliative care, one needs to compare how conventional medicine remains singularly focused on treating the disease. Dr Srinagesh Simha, co-founder and medical director of Karunashraya, a palliative care centre in Bengaluru, explains, 'In medicine, traditionally, the focus most of the time is on cure. A person has a "disease" that needs to be diagnosed, and this must be "cured". Not being able to do so is considered as a "failure". Interventions like surgery, radiation, chemotherapy, medications, etc. are given primacy. Palliative care is transformative because it centres the human experience in all its complexity. For healthcare providers, it invites a deeper, more compassionate approach to care that connects them to their own humanity. For families, it offers a space where grief, love and meaning can coexist, allowing them to face their challenges with more support and understanding. By addressing the whole person, palliative care fosters a sense of dignity, respect and peace that has a profound and lasting impact on everyone involved.'

While the person who is ill suffers the most, the suffering caused by a life-threatening or life-limiting illness also expands to take in the family, companions and guardians. Harmala Gupta, a cancer survivor and founder of CanSupport that provides free home-based palliative care in many parts of North India, explains, 'Caregivers are usually at sea when looking after a patient with a serious illness. They do not know what to expect and how to respond to the constantly shifting needs and moods of their loved one. This is where professional palliative care support can help. Caregivers can be taught simple techniques, like cleaning and bandaging a wound, and be equipped with medications to deal with an emergency. The process of dying must be explained to them. They should also be counselled on how to deal with their own emotions and sensitized to the emotional needs of someone in distress, and how best to respond to strong emotions like anger. If caregivers do not receive support from palliative care professionals, it is likely that the final days of their loved one will become an unbearable burden. This in turn can complicate the process of grieving and can lead to depression and psychological pain.'

All over India, doctors don't generally see pain as a serious problem to be dealt with. It is seen perhaps as a natural concomitant of disease. As patients, we accept it with resignation, though we don't have to. For too long, the fundamental change that is required in this attitude has not happened.

Dr Sushma Bhatnagar, who has moved from AIIMS (Delhi), where she did stellar work on palliative care, to Indraprastha Apollo Hospitals, says, 'Illness doesn't just bring physical pain; it often affects a person emotionally, socially and spiritually as well. Many doctors, however, tend to focus only on physical pain because that's what we're trained to manage. But patients often experience much more – feelings of fear, isolation and uncertainty – that can add to their suffering. It's not just about managing symptoms like pain or shortness of breath, it's also about making sure the person feels supported emotionally, has their social needs met and finds peace spiritually. Treating the whole person is crucial because when you only focus on physical pain, you miss so much of what's going on inside.'

Health-related pain is not only physical, as Dr Cicely Saunders, the founder of the modern palliative care movement, pointed out astutely. For, illness brings with it social stigmas and can cause social pain. It is often expensive and disrupts carefully balanced budgets, causing economic pain. It brings us into contact with complicated and people-unfriendly systems and causes bureaucratic pain. It makes us wonder what we did to deserve the suffering, and if we are religious, this can cause spiritual pain. It rewrites our routine, it undermines our dignity, and this brings psychological pain.

Palliative care seeks to end the reign of total pain. Not just physical pain as we shall see, although when a human being is in acute physical pain, there is nothing more beautiful and more desirable than relief from it. But once that has been dealt with, pain can take many other forms, and alleviating all of them is what palliative care seeks to do.

I understood what this means when I visited Guwahati's Dr. Bhubaneswar Borooah Cancer Institute (part of the Tata Memorial Centre), where the palliative care team had fanned out across the village of Kamalpur when they heard that a carpenter had been ostracized after he was diagnosed with cancer. He was recovering, but the village had shunned him. The abandonment was particularly hard because the carpenter had recently lost his son to suicide. The homecare palliative team went from family to family in the village, assuring them that cancer is not contagious and that there is no reason to shun a man who had lived in their midst all his life. In the end, most people were convinced, and the carpenter was reintegrated into his world. Success for the palliative care team meant not just that their patient was in remission, but also that he had been returned to his place in society and that they had helped end the pain of social ostracism too.

And so palliative care is not just about managing the illness, it does not become relevant only at the end of life and it is not just for the patient. Palliative care also comes in to bring relief from total pain, to share the burden, to lighten the load, to listen to the patient and the caregiver, to suggest solutions and to link you up to others who have the same problems, who have walked the same road and may have some wisdom for you. And if not wisdom, at least an acknowledgement that yes, life can be like this, and we are in this together.

Get Him to Sit Up

Dr Ira Almeida, project director of the palliative care unit at South Goa District Hospital, was in her OPD when she saw a young man on a trolley. He had been brought in by his friend, another young man, who was sitting on the bench across from him. The friend had brought the young man there in his taxi and had carried him into the clinic.

Dr Almeida relates this young man's story to me.

'When he was eight years old, he had gone to some celebration in his school. A large stage had been put up, and when a thunderstorm broke out, he scuttled under the stage, which collapsed on him, and he was paralysed. He told us he had been bed-bound since then. When I was checking him over, I asked him if he could lift his head. He could. We found he had control over the upper half of his body. I asked him to sit up and he said he couldn't. "See, I have this," he said. He had undergone a suprapubic cystostomy, which drains urine from the body. Instead of draining it through the penis, a tube is inserted above the pubic bone because this sometimes does a better job of draining the urine when the bladder is not emptying well. He said, "I have come to have the tube changed. If I sit up, it will get blocked." This was not true, but someone had told him that this might happen or had left him with the impression that this might happen, and so it was now a fixed idea in his head. I told Sudha, the nurse, and Sonali, the occupational therapist on our team: "Your first job is to get him to sit up."'

Dr Almeida continues her story: 'The team persuaded him to let them visit him at his home by saying that they would change his tube themselves. This would spare him the day's journey, and his friend would not have to give up his earnings to bring him to the OPD. When we visited his home, we saw that he was living in quite a terrible condition. He would be lying in a bed in a room all day, staring at the walls. His mother grew and sold vegetables for a living, so she was out most of the day. It took a while for trust to grow but eventually, the team did get him to sit up. The next step was to get him into a wheelchair. Now, no longer bed-bound, he gets about the house and even helps his mother with her work. We wanted to get him out of the house, but the wheelchair would not fit through the door, so we are trying to organize a child's wheelchair so that he can get out to the front of the house. The house does not have a ramp, of course. I am going to try and get one of my builder friends to build a ramp there.'

For Lizzy, a medical social worker, the next goal is to get the young man to start earning. 'He will be making envelopes, which we will get decorated and sell at our office or at Christmas bazaars, wherever we can get them in,' she tells me.

To my mind, this story illustrates many of the most important aspects of palliative care. To begin with, it negates the commonly held myth that palliative care is meant only for those who have cancer, and even within that group, for those who are terminal with just a few weeks or months to live. The young man in this story did not suffer from cancer. He was paralysed and unable to take care of himself independently. Palliative care, therefore, is about any of several life-limiting and life-threatening diseases. Its ambit can take in the infant, the adolescent and the senescent. Its arc can run over decades.

Next, the story illustrates the five main precepts that guide palliative care, which are the principles that also guide – or should guide – medical practice. They are: first, to find ways to increase 'patient autonomy' – to respect the patient as a person; second, to remember 'beneficence' – the call to do good; third, to be guided by the principle of 'non-malfeasance' – to minimize harm in all interventions; fourth, to be directed by practising 'justice' in ensuring the fair use of available resources; and lastly, to demonstrate 'collaboration' – to build an ecosystem of care and involve other professionals in the care of the patient and family.

Patient autonomy requires those who are trying to help someone to ask what she or he wants. The young man's decision was clear and absolute. He preferred to keep lying down in his misery, convinced that he would be worse off sitting up. Now the onus was on the palliative care team to reassure him otherwise and make that happen.

The medical professionals who continue to check over the young man and make sure he is in good health are trying to make a tangible difference. The regularity and dependability of the care all adds up to doing good.

The overall approach is about minimizing harm. Working at the pace of the young man, the team looks for ways to engage his mind and his body while minimizing risks. A bored human being is a human being in distress; a human being in distress is a body in distress too, and that is not a state that can be defined as good health.

By giving the young man the opportunity to make envelopes, fair use is being made of all available resources: Time, effort and money are well utilized to restore confidence and a sense of agency.

In the friend who volunteered to bring him to the hospital, we see the figure of a man who will come to the aid of his fellow beings for no reason other than that they share the same humanity.

The doctor, nurse, therapist and social worker all join to extend multidisciplinary care to the boy and his mother. The ramp will come out of the pocket of someone whose conscience has been prodded by Dr Almeida. And now, the envelopes will be bought by people who understand that it is in our small acts of kindness that we illumine lives. This is palliative care, where to do good becomes its own reward.

Sadly though, most patients aren't fortunate enough to be surrounded by this kind of compassionate care.

Most families don't get the help they need to carry the weight of their circumstances.

A Journey Reimagined

With all this, I now run a thought experiment in my head. My Uncle M was diagnosed with cancer of the larynx. He was to have surgery but was not told, until he woke up, that his voice would be taken from him. After the operation, which was declared a success, he discovered that he would never speak again.

I remember the doctor telling me, 'You speak English at home, no? He doesn't know that the voice box is the larynx? What did he think would happen if we take out the larynx?'

I was angry at the doctor's assumption that words like larynx would be comprehensible to anyone speaking English, at him transferring the blame to our family. I was angry but I was silent because he was a doctor, and he was in charge. My aunt, meanwhile, was making conciliatory sounds because she was aware that she was going to ask him to reduce his surgery fee.

I think now about Uncle M and his life in Konkani, a rich life of expletive songs and Rabelaisian humour.

His English was like his three-piece suit. He wore it when he stepped out. Larynx, pharynx, transection ... These words were not part of his vocabulary. He was told that the cancer would kill him unless he allowed the surgeon to operate. The surgeon operated and Uncle M fell into silence. He lived a half-life after that, coming to parties and wanting to sing, writing out smutty jokes on pieces of paper and watching sadly as people smiled embarrassedly at the asterisks he put in and rolled their eyes. There was no attempt at rehabilitation, no one to ask whether he would like to learn to talk through an electrolarynx. He was supposed to be grateful that he was alive.

I run the same scenario through palliative care now. There would be someone to help Uncle M understand what the surgery would mean. Perhaps someone to prepare him for the idea of an electrolarynx. Speech therapy and perhaps even the palliative care team as an audience for his jokes when they visited. If anything, palliative care is the kind heart of medicine. How much Uncle M would have benefited, how much we all would have benefited from some attempt at going beyond the condition to the person who had the condition, to who he was before and who he would like to be afterwards.

The truth of the matter is that we all need help, and this does not go only for those who are ill. Human civilization is posited on our interdependence. The problem is how that help is offered. Is it offered as a form of charity? Then accepting it requires a posture of subservience. Is it offered as a favour? Then no reliance can be placed on its continuance. Is it offered as a matter of fact, the fact of you, that you are here, that you belong and that you have the right to assistance when you need it? Is it offered to you simply because you are one of the eight-point-something billion people on the planet and so are entitled to just as much as the next human being is?

It's for You and Me

We are unique; we are stardust and primordial energy; we are communities in ourselves with bacteria that feed us and protect us; we are, each one of us, beautifully and spectacularly made with organs that interlock, senses that draw the world in and neurons that sieve and transform that information into the specific thoughts and feelings that make us unique, the one in the many.

But this very intricateness, this poise, and balance is a fragile thing; it is prone to imbalance if subjected to disturbance, showing us how much we need each other.

Human beings are evolutionarily ill-equipped to face the world independently. We've survived and even achieved dominance because we learned how to work together. Everything – from something as basic as language to a system as complicated as democracy – depends on consensus: an agreement on meaning, aims and means; an agreement to work together as a group, each one bringing individual skills and talents to the task at hand. Even as hunter-gatherers, we recognized that we can do much more when we combine forces than when we try to make a go of it alone.

The renowned anthropologist Margaret Mead said that in her mind, the first sign of civilization was finding a healed femur at an ancient site. This meant that the notion of caring had overridden the notion of 'survival of the fittest'. If the man with the broken femur had been left alone, he would have starved to death. That he did not means that someone cared for him, bringing him food and water until the broken bone had healed and he had recovered.

If our civilization amounts to anything, then it must be based on caring for each other. Health is everyone's business, health is everyone's concern – no one gets a pass. If there is anything that demonstrates our interconnectedness, it is the business of health, at once located in the body and in all that surrounds it.

Palliative care concerns all of us, each one of us. As Rosalynn Carter, wife of the late president of the United States Jimmy Carter, once said, 'There are only four kinds of people in the world – those that have been caregivers, those that are caregivers, those who will be caregivers and those who will need caregivers.'

3

The Science and Art of Palliative Care

The term 'palliative care' comes from the Latin word 'pallium' or cloak. It suggests the warmth and protection of such a garment. In its ordinary English sense, it means to make something better by making someone feel better.

At the Cipla Palliative Care Centre, Pune, a comprehensive palliative care centre with inpatient, outpatient and homecare services, I meet Lakshmi, a woman braving the challenges of breast cancer. She began coming to the centre just a month ago, feeling overwhelmed by pain and exhaustion after her surgery. Dr Vivek Nirabhawane, head of clinical services at the centre, is checking on her using a multidimensional assessment tool called the Edmonton Symptom Assessment System that allows patients to rate their symptoms on a scale of 0 to 10. With a smile that lit up her face, Lakshmi shares that her pain has significantly eased. The medication is finally making a difference. Today, she is excited about the group physiotherapy session – a time not just for movement but also for connection. In this space, she finds relief from her muscle stiffness and, equally importantly, a sense of belonging among friends who understand her journey.

When I visit the National Institute of Mental Health and Neurosciences (NIMHANS), Bengaluru, I meet Vishwas, who is dealing with advanced Parkinson's disease. He is accompanied by his devoted wife, and together they face the challenges of daily life. Their son has brought them to the palliative care OPD because Vishwas has been struggling to swallow and is feeling unsteady on his feet. The palliative care team, including a caring occupational therapist, steps in to assess his needs and risks. They patiently teach Vishwas some helpful exercises for his hands and safe swallowing techniques. They even adjust his wheelchair to make him more comfortable and show his family how to safely move him into and out of the chair. And to ease their worries further, the team promises to visit their home next week to check on his progress.

The Science and Art of Palliative Care

At Sukoon Nilaya, an inpatient palliative care centre for all serious illnesses in Mumbai, I meet Rajesh, a forty-five-year-old man on the road to recovery after a stroke. He has been referred from a local hospital, and Dr Leena Gangoli, the palliative care physician at the centre, and her dedicated team are busy teaching Rajesh's wife how to blend his food and serve it in a cup, making mealtime easier for him. The physiotherapist encourages Rajesh to practise buttoning his shirt, helping him regain his independence, one small step at a time.

The problem is that too often palliative care is seen as death-haunted, when it is, in fact, life-affirming. Contrary to mainstream perception, palliative care promises an improved quality of life not just at the end but also from the time one needs it – till the very end.

Dr Sultan Pradhan, founder of the Punyashlok Ahilyadevi Holkar Institute of Head and Neck Cancer, the new ninety-three-bedded facility in South Mumbai, ensures that misperceptions about palliative care as terminal care do not affect his practice. He says,

'I prefer to call the palliative care team the "supportive care team" because it emphasizes what we're really here to do: to support the patient through every stage of their illness, not just at the end. Supportive care is about helping patients manage symptoms, emotional challenges and quality of life throughout their treatment. For head and neck cancer patients, the side effects are often complex – pain, difficulty swallowing and speech issues, for example. Having a supportive care team from the start helps ease these struggles and prevents things from getting worse. By addressing the physical, emotional and social aspects early on, we can reduce distress, improve outcomes and make the whole journey more manageable for both the patient and their caregivers.'

More doctors and patients need to see palliative care as a partner in curative care, not the final chapter. That it is really about helping people live better while they're being treated. To get what palliative care is all about, we need to revisit its roots in easing suffering and focusing on the person, not just the illness. Embracing this focus matters now, more than ever.

A Short History of Palliative Care

The founder of the palliative care movement in the modern world was Dr Cicely Saunders, a six-foot-tall British woman who started out as a nurse during the Second World War. But when she hurt her back, she retrained as a 'lady almoner', a social service worker, in a hospital. It was during this time that she met David Tasma, a terminally ill Polish man, in Archway Hospital, London. Like many of those with incurable cancer, he had been tucked away at the end of the ward, forgotten by the medical establishment that did not want to acknowledge that it had failed to heal him. They fell in love, the girl from Roedean and the dying refugee, and it was the beginning of a revolution in healthcare.

Dr Saunders could see how badly the health system was treating the man she loved and all the others who were dying, and she wanted something better for them, something much better. She wanted a place full of light and hope. She shared her dream with Tasma, and when he died, he left her five hundred pounds, with which she made a beginning. Dr Saunders also saw that if she had to make a real difference in the lives of the terminally ill, she would have to learn how to keep them comfortable and as pain-free as medically possible. So, she trained to become a doctor. It took her nineteen years to realize the dream she had shared with Tasma, but eventually, in 1967, St Christopher's Hospice, London, opened its doors to the public.

In the early 1960s, another female doctor, in the United States this time, Dr Elisabeth Kübler-Ross, began to walk to the end of the hospital's wards, where she would talk to the dying who had been put there, tucked out of sight and abandoned. These conversations eventually ended up in her devising the stages of grief that come with a diagnosis of a terminal illness: denial, anger, bargaining, depression and acceptance. She would write a series of books, including the path-breaking *On Death and Dying*.

Dr Saunders had had some experience of watching the suffering of someone she loved without being able to do much to ameliorate it. And perhaps the ambition of her revolution also arose from her stereoscopic view of her patients. Her training enabled her to see them from three distinct perspectives – from the points of view of a social worker, a nurse and a doctor.

From these perspectives, Dr Saunders challenged the usual definition of pain, which in medicine is still seen only as the distress call of the neuron. She devised the notion of 'total pain', asking us all to look at pain as a matrix. She pointed out that someone who is ill might feel physical pain, true, but that isn't the sum total of the distress. There is also the financial distress that comes with worries about paying bills or loss of income; the social discomfort that one might feel if one has a disease that is stigmatized, as AIDS continues to be; the psychological pain that comes with all of the above, to which may be added the loss of one's agency, the need to depend on others and the lack of dignity; and no less is the spiritual agony when one wonders why one is suffering when the whole world, it seems, is in good health and what one's beliefs mean.

Dr Saunders would revisit the notion of 'total pain' again and again, and each time she would raise the bar for palliative care. To her, it was not enough to ease physical discomfort. The palliative care team had to ease all these various pains, working at any number of levels and bringing all available resources to bear.

Reflecting on my conversation with the late Dr Robert Twycross, a pioneer in palliative care and symptom management, who graduated from the University of Oxford's medical college in 1965 and later worked as a clinical researcher under Dr Cicely Saunders, I am reminded of Dr Saunders' vision – not only to build an evidence base but also to champion the global spread of modern palliative care.

Dr Twycross's writings, including his work on the *Oxford Textbook of Palliative Medicine*, have played a pivotal role in making palliative care a key part of modern healthcare. His approach and ideas on advancing holistic approaches to care, addressing not only physical pain but also emotional, psychological and spiritual suffering have helped shape the thinking around caring for people with serious illnesses.

Palliative Care in India

In India, modern palliative care, it is generally agreed, started when Dr Luis Jose DeSousa (fondly known as Dr Luzito) founded the first hospice, Shanti Avedna Sadan, on Mount Mary Road in Bandra, Mumbai, in 1986 and invited Dr Cicely Saunders to inaugurate it. But her husband's illness prevented that from happening. However, she remained a staunch ally and sent a message of congratulations when Dr DeSousa organized the first international hospice conference in India in 1991, saying she had followed his progress 'with admiration'. If she had made it, perhaps she would have been able to inaugurate the Goa branch too, which opened a fortnight later in an Indo-Portuguese house in Loutolim.

Dr DeSousa shares with me when I meet him in his clinic in Mumbai that there is no limit to caring. 'That is why palliative care must start early with non-communicable diseases, like cancer. Many patients may be lucky and go into remission. But when the cancer comes back, we can only manage it; we can rarely cure it,' he says.

And this management is caring. With love and professional commitment, for as long as it takes.

The early 1990s saw the seeds of palliative care in India take root. The formation of pain and palliative care societies in Guwahati, Calicut and Ahmedabad; the setting up of palliative care centres like the Cipla Palliative Care Centre in Pune and Karunashraya in Bengaluru; homecare services in

Delhi through CanSupport as well as the formation of the Indian Association of Palliative Care (IAPC). All these nurtured the movement over the next few decades, with doctors in several cancer hospitals providing palliative care as well as advocacy to their patients, and community-based organizations like Pallium India serving patients and their families in Thiruvananthapuram.

The momentum has led up to the Government of India launching the National Palliative Care Programme (NPCP) in 2012 as part of the National Health Mission to enable states to receive funding for setting up palliative care services at the district level. It is heartening that several states, such as Kerala, Maharashtra, Tamil Nadu and Karnataka, have adopted policies to expand palliative care, while other states, such as Goa, have plans to do the same.

Prakash Fernandes, who heads palliative care partnerships at the Cipla Foundation and has been instrumental in strengthening and launching over thirty such projects across India, says, 'It's exciting how dynamically palliative care is finding its place within the healthcare system. This expansion is deeply rooted in creative collaboration – from integrating palliative care into public health initiatives to engaging local communities, leveraging technology, defining quality standards and respecting the unique needs of each health setup.'

While there are many efforts to increase access to palliative care, the stakeholders in the movement in India have had to struggle – and struggle long and hard – even for something as basic as access to a drug that has been providing effective relief from extreme pain across the world for well over a century: morphine.

No More Suffering

It may not be surprising that many of the palliative care professionals today have their roots in anaesthesiology and the setting up of pain clinics. We need to remember, always, that much of what palliative care can do – and should do – begins with the end of physical pain. Pain of the kind that cancer, for instance, produces, is all-encompassing. It will not allow you to think, it will not allow you to assess your life or make a bucket list.

Pain control is one of the first and most important tasks in palliation and the hero of palliation, morphine, is almost as old as the history of medicine. Morphine, an alkaloid found in opium, is one of the most powerful pain relievers known to humanity. Opium has several alkaloids, including codeine and morphine. The latter, first extracted from opium resin in 1803, is the gold standard for pain relief. However, morphine's dark twin dogs its steps. Opium, with its bad reputation, makes life difficult for morphine, which has multiple uses in the world of medicine.

A native of Central and Eastern Europe, the poppy grows pretty much where human beings plant it. When the velvety petals of *Papaver somniferum* fall off, leaving behind the seedpod, slits are made on its surface. Latex begins to ooze and is allowed to dry overnight. This is then collected and dried. For centuries, it was used chiefly as a medicine. It helped with the pain, eased coughing and soothed babies. Ibn Sina, the tenth-century Persian physician, knew about it; it is mentioned in Ayurvedic texts too. It has been grown in India at least since the tenth century CE. As Amitav Ghosh writes in his magnificent book, *Smoke and Ashes: A Writer's Journey through Opium's Hidden Histories,* 'Simply put, opium is perhaps the oldest and most powerful medicine known to man.'

Ghosh's book does a remarkable job of outlining opium's ever-changing role in human history. Indian farmers, he tells us, grew poppy alongside other food crops, at the edges of their fields. When the British East India Company discovered the huge amount of money that was to be made by producing and thrusting the drug into China and India, it forced farmers to cultivate opium. The poppy is a thirsty crop. It needs much labour and manure. And so, very few families in India could afford to grow only poppy, yet that was what the British demanded they do.

But by now opium was no longer just a medicine. It was being used as a recreational drug and started thousands on the road to addiction. Everyone from the upper classes who wanted a mind-altering experience to the labouring classes who wanted relief from the pain of extreme physical labour needed their opium pipes. This is the origin of the bad name opium was given.

The British have left us with a complicated legacy in the matter of opium. It was a cash crop – *the* cash crop – that made fortunes for the East India Company first, for the British Crown thereafter, and they would go to war, if necessary, to protect their drug peddling.

Until very recently, colonial-era laws prevailed, and access to morphine in India did not fall under the purview of the health ministry but came under the Department of Revenue. It is not expensive, nor is it in short supply. Much of the legally grown opium in the world comes from India. Most of it is exported and ends up in the United States and Western Europe, which naturally have much better figures for pain control, leaving 96 per cent of patients in India in need of pain relief suffering, according to the 2017 Lancet Commission report on palliative care.

Binod Hariharan, chairperson of Pallium India, explains: 'One of Pallium's major achievements was the amendment of the Narcotic Drugs and Psychotropic Substances Act, which originated during British times and was allowed to remain unchanged. Opium was a cash crop, and so it came under the Department of Revenue. But the end product, morphine, is a medical product that is to be used for health. However, there was no conversation between the health sector and the bureaucrats making the original Act. At that time, there was very little training in pain relief. That morphine and opioids were important analgesics was left out of the Act. This meant that those who actually needed it had no access to it. In 2014, after nearly eighteen years of work, the Act was amended, and now there is a single law that governs access to morphine across the country. But individual state governments must be made aware of this change and its benefits for patients. Their bureaucratic apparatus has to be changed. They need to know how this would be good for patients and must incorporate it into palliative care programmes.'

Pallium India's founder, Dr Rajagopal, emphasizes that this is important not just at the end of life but also during treatment. 'After all, treating chronic pain is a basic part of being a good doctor. If we don't use tools like morphine when they're needed, we're not doing our job – we're causing unnecessary suffering,' he says

Dr Rajagopal recalls his journey into palliative care. 'There were no other doctors in my family. But when I got the required marks and secured the seat, my father said: "Well, why don't you do that?" And so I became a doctor.'

However, he attributes his interest in palliative medicine to certain memories that he has carried with him. 'As a medical student, I was a day scholar for a while, and when I would go back home, I would hear loud screams, literal howls of torment. They came from a home not far from mine. A distant cousin of mine had cancer; it had metastasized – there were nodules all over his body. The doctors had sent him home saying there was nothing more they could do. He knew I was a medical student, so he asked if I would come and see him. I did and he asked me if there was anything I could do to help him. I couldn't. I was only a student and I had no idea what to do. I made my escape and never visited him again. He died in acute suffering. I think his spirit came to live in me. But all through my medical education, I was not aware of suffering. The best professors were dismissive of it. They just did not see it. Perhaps I knew I was running away from it, building protective walls around myself against the memory of my cousin's pleading.'

This deeply personal failure became the foundation for transformative change. It led Dr Rajagopal to set up Pallium India in 2003 and the Thiruvananthapuram Institute of Palliative Care (TIPS) in 2006. These together work relentlessly, not just in Kerala but also at the national level, to put pain management and palliative care on the national medical radar.

Dignity for Every Life

It has been a long road that patients, families and medical professionals have walked, and through it all, one idea has been paramount: that the patient should be spared all pain – pain of any kind.

Take a moment to let that sink in.

The patient should be spared pain of any kind.

I know. You're thinking what I too thought at the beginning of this project: How can a doctor do all of this alone? Manage complex symptoms, navigate difficult conversations, create a nurturing environment for healing, account for the economic situation of the family, relieve doubts about the disease and the prognosis, help with the stigma the family may face, link them up to others who have been through this …?

The answer is simple. The doctor isn't supposed to do it all. The doctor is a doctor and has a doctor's role to play in the total pain alleviation programme. The responsibility is not the doctor's alone. There is an interdisciplinary team, and once the work is spread out across this team of committed people, each one focused on the goal of making things work out for patients and their families, it is not undoable.

In fact, it is very doable.

As Mahatma Gandhi said, 'A small body of determined spirits fired by an unquenchable faith in their mission can alter the course of history.'

4

An Interdisciplinary Approach to Healthcare

Most palliative care, without being called that, probably takes place within the confines of the family in India. One often hears tales of heroism, but the toll on a family or on the person who is appointed as a caregiver can be terrible. Love wears away under the strain of bedpans and midnight dashes to the hospital. Much of this is assigned to the woman of the family, generally without so much as a by-your-leave. The mother, the wife, the daughter, the sister – she is expected to nurture and provide care, feed, soothe, clean up and take the brunt of despair and frustration that can make the afflicted person weep or lash out.

When all of this is done well, it isn't noticed. The patient is quiet, clean and generally grateful. But when something goes wrong – a bedsore shows up because a bedridden old woman was not turned often enough, or an opportunistic infection develops because a child insists on eating street food – the caregiver is blamed. This adds insult to injury.

The whole aim of the palliative care movement is to bring the patient and the beleaguered caregiver into a support system of caring so that there can be a shared responsibility for the sick person. There are many people who must bring different skills to bear in the situation.

The Doctor

Palliative care is no single person's responsibility. It is a team effort, and each member of the team plays their part in providing the wraparound comfort, the 360-degree solution that palliative care demands as every patient's entitlement. The doctor is obviously one of the team members. Perhaps the doctor's position in the team can be compared to the position of the prime minister in a cabinet of ministers, *primus inter pares* – first among equals.

By law, only doctors can prescribe morphine or opioids, and so they are in charge of alleviating physical pain.

A doctor's responsibility is to ease suffering, for healing can only begin once pain is addressed. However, doctors can face challenges in managing pain effectively, including the need for accurate assessment, individualized treatment plans and balancing medication side effects with therapeutic benefits.

Dr Manjula B.V., trustee of the Pain Relief and Palliative Care Society (PRPCS), Hyderabad, says, 'I've seen patients come in screaming, begging us to end their suffering. When we finally bring the pain under control and they have a good night's sleep without pain, it's like they return to themselves. I've seen patients go from barely being able to sit up to smiling, talking and laughing with their loved ones, like they are back from the kingdom of pain, able to enjoy the simple things again. Witnessing that shift is one of the most rewarding parts of being a doctor – it's not just about relieving pain but also about helping patients reclaim their sense of normalcy and joy.'

Effective pain management can completely transform a patient's experience. It takes them from feeling overwhelmed and trapped in a vice of pain to regaining control over their lives. But the doctor cannot do it alone.

Dr Jayarajan Ponissery, Medical Director of the Cipla Palliative Care Centre, explains, 'Palliative care is truly an intersectional speciality. It draws from various fields like ethics, economics and public policy because the care we provide goes beyond just the physical aspects of illness. As palliative care professionals, we need to think about the bigger picture like ensuring the patient's dignity, navigating difficult decisions with families and understanding the financial and systemic impacts of care.'

He adds, 'Today, in our team meeting, we discussed a patient who wants to go back home, outside of Pune, but his family wants him to stay on at the centre. We decided that the social work team would support both the patient and his wife and son to jointly discuss their fears and hopes. The nurses will support the family by teaching them how they can care for the patient at home with diet and exercise, and how to prevent bedsores and clean his wounds. The physicians will try to bring down his pain and nausea. We will regroup tomorrow to review how the patient and family members feel about the situation and hopefully agree on a plan for the patient to go home in a safe manner, acceptable to the family, knowing that they can reach out to us at any time.'

An Interdisciplinary Approach to Healthcare

No single person can be an expert in so many different fields and doctors must learn to rely on each other and on the strengths of others.

'The Medical Council of India recognized the need for this specialized branch of palliative medicine in 2010, and the first specialist MD in palliative medicine started at TMH, Mumbai, in 2012,' says Dr Mary Ann Muckaden, a strong advocate of palliative care. She adds, 'The three-year curriculum is designed to help these professionals to provide comprehensive care to patients with serious illness and support patients and families to be better prepared as they seek treatment. Added to this is the development of a Diplomate of National Board (DNB) course in palliative medicine. However, there are very few MD/DNB palliative care doctors graduating each year, so we need to have six-week training programmes with direct work experience for MBBS doctors to enable them to provide good quality care.'

In an interview with *Civil Society* magazine, Dr Gayatri Palat, an anaesthesiologist who is the trustee of PRPCS in Hyderabad and has had remarkable success with incorporating palliative care at the district level in Telangana, said, 'It's not just about having a doctor. The doctor's role is, I would say, maybe 25 per cent of what alleviating suffering is about.'[3]

But in a hospital setting, someone has to be answerable to management. 'Someone needs to be head of the department,' says Dr Veronique Dinand, head of the palliative care department at Bai Jerbai Wadia Hospital for Children, Mumbai, 'and so, I am the head, but actually if you look at it from the patient's point of view, there is not a single member of the team who is dispensable. Each one contributes their bit. I deal with the physical symptoms and some of the psychological worry associated with a sick child simply because a white coat and a stethoscope can make the parents feel that some help is at hand. But if we are to deal with the total pain of the patient, then every member of the team must do their bit.'

And then, out of the ordinary ways of palliative care, sometimes a doctor may turn detective. When I visited Karunashraya in Bengaluru, Dr Srinagesh Simha told me a story: 'A patient told us she had been married in the past and had two children. Then she fell in love with someone else and walked out on her family. Now she wanted to reconnect with her children. Her husband, she knew, had relocated to Delhi and the children had grown up there. This seemed like a job for the detectives. But I had a friend visit me and he asked: "Why so morose?" I told him what I needed, and he said his nephew was a lawyer in Delhi and he would put him on the job.

'This enterprising man checked with the Bar Council of India, where he found that the husband had died but he did a little more digging and found that the son was also a lawyer, and he got hold of his telephone number. So we called the son and told him about his mother's dying wishes. At first, he got a shock because he had been told his mother was dead. We asked if he would come and see her. He refused but agreed to talk to her on the phone. So mother and son had a conversation, and she could make some peace with her past.'

There is so much that I love about this story. A doctor understanding a patient's dilemma without judging her. A doctor wanting to help a patient with her world rather than with just her symptoms. A doctor seeking out children so that a patient could find some form of closure.

There are truly no silos in palliative care.

And for the doctor, too, it can be a transformative experience. Dr Eric Borges, honorary chairperson of the King George V Memorial Trust and cardiologist at the Bombay Hospital Institute of Medical Sciences that set up 'Sukoon Nilaya' – Mumbai's first inclusive palliative care inpatient centre – tells me, 'Nothing in your medical training can prepare you for the lived experience of palliative care. It requires no small measure of unlearning, which is an exercise in humility; it then asks you to learn how to respond to a patient in toto, to look beyond the condition presented to the person as a whole; and finally, each day brings with it a new raft of learning because disease may be predictable in symptoms and patterns but people are never predictable.'

The Nurse

'Nursing is the key to palliative care. Doctors come in and out, we mean well, most of the time hopefully, but nurses are always there,' says Dr Pamela Hutton from the United Kingdom, who first came to India in 1991 to help Dr M.T. Bhatia start palliative care at the Gujarat Cancer & Research Institute, Ahmedabad.

Yashodha Dharkar, chairperson of the Indore Cancer Foundation, says, 'We would benefit from the guidance of chronic pain specialists and nurses skilled in assessing pain. Nurses spend more time with patients and are readily available to respond to their needs. By systematically documenting pain scores, nurses lay the foundation for comprehensive and effective pain relief. Skilled chronic pain specialists are adept at using combinations of medications, administered "by the clock", to ensure consistent pain relief. A valuable lesson can be drawn from the late Dr Robert Twycross, a legendary figure in pain management. His bedside teaching emphasized a comprehensive approach, involving carefully calibrated pharmaceutical combinations. He would adapt these regimens over time, sometimes adding or subtracting medications or employing synergistic drugs to achieve optimal relief.'

Nurses are a constant presence in the ward. To the patient, they seem to be the ones in control of the pain medication. They are the ones who have to find a vein for the injection or IV. Theirs is the first face you see when you surface from anaesthesia. The *CBS Handbook on Pain & Palliative Care*[4] emphasizes that nurses can significantly contribute to training caregivers in managing the long-term needs of patients. They also help bridge the communication gap between physicians, patients and caregivers.

Sister Hanife MacGamwell, an oncology palliative care nurse specialist who has worked in clinics across the world, feels that nurses are a hugely underutilized resource and need to be supported better. 'The curriculum needs to have more hands-on training. Palliative care training needs to encourage and demonstrate to nurses the importance of bedside nursing care, empowering nurses to believe that quality nursing skills are equally important to manage the well-being of patients and caregivers.'

Palliative care nursing is different. While riding with a CanSupport palliative homecare team in Delhi, Sr Sini, the homecare nurse, helps me learn the difference: 'This is more work than we ever do in hospitals. There we catheterize or cannulate or inject or bandage and we move on. Patients in a big ward are often referred to by bed numbers or procedures –

"The hysterectomy wants a bedpan" or "Bed 5 reports breathing problems". Here we meet our patients again and again over time. We see them at home. We meet the family and so a bond is formed. This means that nursing becomes an intense experience because as you get to know the patient better, the patient is getting worse, and you are witness to that degeneration.'

And if doctors are in perennial short supply across India, it might be good to remember that Indian nurses are now valued for their skill and their work ethic across the world. This means that we are running out of nurses, and many teams must make do with nursing aides.

In Guwahati, Assam, I meet Sudip Rudrapaul, a nursing supervisor. He worked for three years at the Cipla Palliative Care Centre in Pune and then moved to Assam to be closer to his parents who live in Tripura. He has been providing palliative care training through the End-of-Life Nursing Education Consortium (ELNEC) project. He tells me, 'Dealing with death and dying is the hardest part of my job. For other nurses, a patient has an appendectomy, they recover, they go home in good health – that is how the nurse proves their effectiveness at their job. For me,

I see the patient return again and again, and at times there is a deterioration and things turn negative. In the clinical support I provide, whether it's managing pain through medication, adjusting treatment plans or offering emotional comfort, I ensure that the patient feels cared for and seen in their most vulnerable moments. And then, when the patient smiles, I hold on to that smile. It is my reward.'

On all the home visits I attended, it was the nurses who seemed to humanize the entire experience. Sometimes they would call a hesitant child out of a corner and coo over her new dress. Sometimes they would pop into the kitchen and exchange recipes and hints. It turned what is sometimes a fraught business into a human encounter. I remember going on a home visit in Goa. We were visiting Ramesh who was once a hotelier. He'd had a stroke which paralysed half his body, and he had been bedridden ever since.

Ramesh's body is skeletal. His continued existence is either a study in the human body's determination to live, or a triumph of the care he is receiving, or both. This time his mouth needs to be cleaned, and a toothbrush is wrapped in a cloth and dipped in water. He cooperates but clamps down once in a while as if this is a signal of his resistance and his presence; he is alive, he isn't to be pitied or forgotten. The nurse understands. She will not give up. She cajoles, coaxes, mock-scolds and finally coos in triumph when Ramesh lets her finish.

'What will you cook for me when I come next?' the nurse asks jokingly.

'Ask my wife!' Ramesh says.

Everyone in the room dissolves into laughter.

The Social Worker

'If we are to take palliative care to the next level,' says Dr Vidya Viswanath, assistant professor of palliative medicine at Homi Bhabha Cancer Hospital & Research Centre, Visakhapatnam, 'It can only be by looking at each individual case as a new beginning. We may be able to take some of our learnings from our history but if they become a formula, then we lose sight of the reason that we are here: this patient with this disease at this stage in its progression in this social situation with this family in this house.'

The specificities of these patients call for help from a social worker.

'I once asked one of my residents to find out how many of our patients did not know their date of birth. Turns out it was nearly 21 per cent,' says Dr Rajendra Badwe, former director of TMC If patients lack even basic identification details, how can they effectively access or benefit from plans and schemes designed for their care?

For many of those who turn up at public hospitals the size of TMC, poverty is the unspoken complication. For the majority of India – those beneath the poverty line and many above it – an illness can be an economic disaster too. 'If the wage-earner falls ill,' says Dr Armida Fernandez of the Romila Palliative Centre, Mumbai, 'It has a ripple effect across the family. Even across generations. Children may be pulled out of school. The spouse may have to find work and the wage-earner experiences a loss in status, an erasure of identity as provider for the family.'

Dr Manjula B.V. of PRPCS, Hyderabad, agrees: 'Even if treatment is free at a hospital, there are always incidental expenses. First, the cost of travel. Then, the cost of staying in the district or the city for the caregiver if the patient is admitted to the hospital. Then it is often the case that some medicines will be prescribed that are not available at the hospital and must be bought outside. And there is also the loss of income to be factored in.'

This is where the social worker steps in. Many of the larger hospitals have social workers on their staff. TMC, for instance, started a Social Services Cell as early as 1950 to help the poor deal with what Rumana Hamied, director of the Veha Foundation and a passionate advocate of palliative care, calls the 'tsunami that is cancer'. Today, the social worker is also an integral part of the palliative care team; the mandate is not restricted to helping the patient or the family find the funds for treatment. At TMC, they've introduced a special team called 'Kevats' – essentially patient navigators who act like guides through the maze of the hospital. Imagine having a trusted companion by your side from the moment you step in, helping you find your way through endless floors, departments and confusing medical jargon. Later in the book, I dive deeper into this unique model.

In Hyderabad, I went on a homecare visit with Ravi Kumar, a social worker at PRPCS. He tells me the story of the family we are going to visit. 'One of the children has cerebral palsy. We thought this was a challenge because the father is a daily-wage labourer and the family lives in a hut. Then we found out that the father is an alcoholic and abusive. One day we got a call from the mother of the child saying that her husband was forcing her to abandon the child. She has three other children to take care of. She is also prone to depression. She has sought help and was given a prescription, but the antidepressants make her drowsy. She can't stay awake. Because she sleeps, one of the elder children must stay at home to look after the youngest. The eldest, a fourteen-year-old boy, had dropped out of school to find work to support the family; the third had followed suit.'

It is a disease-haunted family that needs rehabilitation at so many levels. 'First, we decided that the mother and child needed respite care, so we brought them to the hospice. This allowed the mother to recover from the emotional and physical strain, while the child could receive specialized care in a safe environment,' says Kumar. 'Then we set up a chain of donors to supply them with dry rations and school fees. This handled some of the economic problems and at least the children could return to school.'

The Counsellor

The next member of the team is a mental health professional, a psychologist or a counsellor. There are many names by which they go but their function is to provide a listening ear that is trained for and attuned to the needs of patients and their families. In some organizations, the social workers are trained to provide counselling support to patients and their families.

Patients in the medical system are often silenced by the nature of the system. The doctor is busy, there are so many other patients waiting, there is so much noise in the hospital, there are so many questions, but it doesn't seem right to be asking them. And even when it is all sorted out, the patient has a diagnosis, the medication schedule has been explained, the side effects have been covered, Google has been consulted, there is a question that keeps coming back: Why me?

'When they hear the diagnosis, if it is a dreaded disease or a condition that cannot be cured, there is often blankness. They don't know how to respond, what to think,' says Poojitha Kandikanthi, a social worker at PRPCS. The mental health professional's role is not to give the patient the 'right' response or answers but to guide them in exploring their own feelings and solutions. The focus is on empowering the patient to facilitate self-discovery, growth and healing.

'Most of the time I am silent. I listen,' says Sameer Cuncolkar, who works as a counsellor-cum-social worker at the Goa Medical College and Hospital. 'It is good for them to talk. They often want to say: "I led a good life. I had no bad habits. I worked hard all my life. Why am I suffering like this when nothing happens to corrupt politicians?" There is no answer to that but airing the question can help ease the pain of feeling singled out for suffering.'

The counsellors are trained to identify the feelings of patients and reflect them back so as to enable

An Interdisciplinary Approach to Healthcare

patients to find their own answers to some of the questions and find their own coping mechanisms.

The mental health professional must contend with how a simple wish has morphed into an impossible dream. A patient may say he would like to go down to the river and have a bath as he did for so many years and then go to the temple. But this may never happen now, or not quite as normally as it used to happen. The counsellor must communicate this fact gently – with honesty, but also with reasonable, realistic hope.

'We ask them to set achievable goals. To go back to the temple is an achievable goal. To have a bath by the river is an achievable goal. It cannot be turned into the everyday occurrence that it was, but we break it down into simpler goals and the patient has the satisfaction of knowing that everyone is working on what is important to them,' says Barbara Maria da Silva, counsellor at the NGO Novi Survat, a children's palliative care organization in Goa.

I think also of the time I walked down a ward with Dr Babita Varkey, director, clinical services at Karunashraya. In the last bed lay a young man in his late twenties. His father is a construction worker who had lost his wife to cancer. His son powered his way through with education and became a civil engineer.

Then cancer appeared in his sinuses and metastasized into his brain. He lost vision and movement after the operation and is now bed-bound. His father has retreated from this double tragedy into alcoholism. There is a sister, but she is also estranged.

There is a quietness about the young man, a resignation. A huge bump on the right side of his head looks ominous. 'The doctors have explained that the prognosis is not good. If the tumour pushes down, he could have a series of strokes and die,' Dr Varkey says. She bends over and talks to him. 'He is conscious about who he is and what is happening, but he often loses sense of time and place, so we have to keep reorienting him every so often.

'One night he could not sleep and was talking to the nurse. He said he had drunk and smoked a lot and had done other terrible things for which he feels he is being punished.'

At one level, the body is the only home the self knows. It is generally seen as a good home. So long as it obeys the directions of the mind and absorbs the damage done by living, we accept its marvellous intricacies as 'normal'. In other words, we take our bodies for granted when we are healthy. Then, one day, the body lets us down. Neurons misfire and even walking demands our entire attention. A secretion ceases somewhere inside the body and fatigue becomes a constant companion. A lump appears, a sense fails, a smooth flow is constricted. This is our common lot, one that we share not just with humanity but also with all complicated life forms of many cells and organs and systems. The difference is that we can feel pity for ourselves unlike wild things that, as D.H. Lawrence tells us through his poem 'Self-Pity', never feel any: *'A small bird will drop frozen dead from a bough without ever having felt sorry for itself.'*

Our problem is that as humans we have enough self-consciousness to know that we are sick and enough temporal consciousness to hark back to the time without sickness and to wish for a life resumed in health.

The Rehabilitation Specialists

If there is a human attribute that we only notice when it has been denied to us, it is dignity. This is an elusive concept because it is so specific to cultural contexts and depends on what one has been used to. But there are some elements common to us all, and physical independence seems to be paramount. To get out of and into bed unaided, to be able to walk, to be alone for a while without raising undue alarm, to attend to one's body in the privacy of a toilet, to not be a burden on anyone, to have control of one's own time, to sleep when one wants to and wake up when one chooses, to cook for oneself and to feed others, to go each day to one's place of worship or to meet a friend, to communicate one's thoughts and feelings to others, to have a conversation that is not about illness, to go back to work and earn a living, to drape oneself in a sari …

These are a sampling of what patients across the country told me that dignity meant to them. In some of these you may feel a resonance somewhere, a feeling of 'Yes, yes, I agree'; in others you will hear the pangs of loss and see how they are memories of what the patient could once do and took for granted.

This is where the speech therapist, the occupational therapist and the physiotherapist come in. When I visit the Homi Bhabha Cancer Hospital & Research Centre in Visakhapatnam, I find Dr Vidya Viswanath, has organized a show-and-tell with the occupational therapist, Subhasmita. The latter had complained that the doctors on the team were not referring patients to her, and Dr Viswanath rightly assumed that this might simply be a matter of doctors not knowing how an occupational therapist might be able to help their patients. (In comparison, speech therapy and physiotherapy seem self-explanatory.) The occupational therapist brings up ways of helping the patients recover their lost sense of dignity. Does a patient have a tremor in their hands? Here is a weighted cup to steady those hands. Is the patient paraplegic? Here are the ways in which the patient can move from a bed to a chair or vice versa. *Send them to me*, she seems to be saying, *and let me help them help themselves*.

At the Romila Palliative Care Centre, Mumbai, I attend a meeting of the Parkinson's Disease Support Group run by a young psychologist, Riddhi Patel, and a neuro-physiotherapist, Kalpana Suresh. At the time of writing this book, they work for the Parkinson's Disease and Movement Disorder Society, started by Dr Bhim Singhal, head of neurology at Bombay Hospital, in 2002. Parkinson's disease brings with it a heavy burden – both for the person affected by it and for the family. The disease is a degenerative one and, many decades after it was first identified, the cause is still unclear. The idea here is to help patients live with and manage their symptoms.

'It is a disease that manifests mostly in the sixth and seventh decades of life,' says Kalpana Suresh. 'There is early onset Parkinson's, which is showing up more and more now after COVID-19. Those patients have a tough time. Many lose their jobs. Some have just married and cannot cope.'

'The disease is different for each person,' Suresh explains, 'so there isn't a single, inflexible approach that can work for everyone. We have worked on a rehabilitation model that our CEO, Dr Maria Barretto, presented in 2023 at the WHO Congress on Parkinson's Disease in Barcelona, which won us wide acclaim.'

'The psychological problems are exacerbated by loneliness and withdrawal,' adds Riddhi Patel. 'There is a stigma attached because the degeneration can be marked not just by mobility issues but also by a change in facial expressions. So, we have to provide a holistic rehabilitation programme, including physiotherapy, of course, but also self-expression, art and dance, yoga, and speech therapy.'

Count the number of therapists you will need to provide a full bouquet to people afflicted with different ailments. These things can multiply, depending on what happens to you. My friend, the painter Jehangir Sabavala, had an operation when a lesion was found in his throat. When he recovered, I remember him telling me about a therapist who came to help him learn to swallow again. Truly, palliative care is an intersectional speciality.

These roles – therapists, counsellors, facilitators – often overlap, and sometimes, mental health professionals will find themselves doing the work of social workers and nurses will find themselves in the position of the quiet listener who allows the patient or the caregiver to unburden themselves.

The Support Team and Volunteers

It is possible to add other elements to this mix. Palliative care is a palette of colours that can be blended endlessly and inventively as long as the patient and their family is kept front and centre; the entire team works together for them.

At the Cipla Palliative Care Centre, Pune, the atmosphere feels less like a hospital and more like that of a home. I see patients and their families chatting away with the support staff, whom they informally call *mama*s (uncle) and *maushi*s (aunt), like they were old friends. I watch a maushi joking with a patient's daughter as they tidy up the bed together, sharing observations about the latest Marathi TV serial. In that small moment, it hits me – the mamas and maushis aren't just caretakers, they represent an extended family, the kind who listens to your worries, shares a laugh with you and makes everything feel just a little lighter. I see how this care isn't just about medicine; it's about making people feel, seen and held.

At every palliative care facility I visit, I see care expand far beyond the doctors and nurses. It's there, in the little, often unnoticed moments: the security guard offering everyone a warm smile as he holds the door open; the driver waiting patiently, making sure families feel looked after during the long rides; and the administrative team greeting everyone with genuine kindness, treating paperwork like it's their own family member's case. It's these small acts that really stand out. The way they ask, 'How are you doing?'

or quietly offer a helping hand when someone looks overwhelmed – it makes all the difference when you know that no matter how tough things get, there's a whole team of people who've got your back, ready to take care of you in every little way.

And then there are the volunteers, the unsung heroes of palliative care. They are the quiet pillars standing by patients and their families, giving everything without expecting anything in return. Many of them have been through it themselves – they've either survived serious illnesses or lost someone close – so they know what this moment felt like. They remember feeling scared, confused and alone. That they have walked this way makes their presence a validation. 'You can get there,' they say without having to say it, 'You can make it through. I did. I'm here.'

All for One: A Case Study

When I first started visiting the Wadia Hospital for Children in Mumbai, I kept coming back, drawn to learn something new from a member of the hospital's vibrant palliative care team. Watching them go about their work felt like witnessing a symphony in motion, with each person playing a part, creating a powerful blend of care and compassion that hits you straight in the heart.

The head of the paediatric Palliative and Supportive Care Unit, Dr Veronique Dinand, who pulls this all together, was born in France but is now the proud possessor of an Indian passport. In 2017, she began to work in palliative care and came to Wadia Hospital in 2019. 'Wadia is the largest charitable children's hospital. It caters to lower- and middle-income group patients so we see a lot of chronic issues, many life-limiting illnesses,' she tells me.

The team has grown steadily: three nurses (one for home care and two on the wards), three counsellors, two social workers, two psychosocial consultants and a doctor on home care. The work goes as deep as it goes wide to give all-around support to each child and every family.

Dr Dinand believes that the demands of taking care of a sick child are intense, and while she plans the care for her patients, she has to watch out for the well-being of her team. She says, 'Many of these children will have to live with these conditions for the rest of their lives. Some can be life-altering; some can be life-limiting.

We try to help with more than just medical solutions because pain is more than just a physical symptom.'

She adds, 'Palliative care requires a real connection between us and the patient. But because of this very real connection, losing a patient can be difficult. It is difficult in all medicine, but if you are a surgeon or working in an emergency ward, you encounter a patient for a very short period of time. Then the next body is wheeled in. Here we have been in contact for a while, and we know a lot about the patient, the family and the situation. This is why the palliative care team meets every Wednesday morning at 10 a.m. to talk about the things that have mattered, the good news and the bad news. Sometimes there is even an attachment to the family after the death of the patient. This is a meeting in which we support each other, reflect on our own feelings, and share our processes without judgement.'

It's incredible how Dr Dinand has built the team creatively and thoughtfully to meet the medical as well as emotional aspects of care. 'We had plenty of books and toys for children,' says Dr Dinand, 'but we didn't have the budget for a librarian, till a grant from the estate of the painter Mehlli Gobhai made it possible.' And thus, Keith D'Souza joined the team at Wadia Hospital. I walk with D'Souza through the wards. (Since many of the children cannot visit the library, the library visits them.) D'Souza carries a bag of books and sits by each bedside, reading out a story in Marathi or Hindi. The happiness of children is addictive. Watching D'Souza enter the cancer ward is a treat. The kids set up a cry of welcome, calling him *dada* (elder brother) or *kaka* (uncle) and even *azoba* (grandfather). 'My reward is when a child forgets their pain or their worries for a moment and points out some detail in an illustration, something I have missed,' says D'Souza.

One afternoon, I find myself attending a Christmas party, organized by the social worker Savio Ponnachan, who also manages the volunteers. On this day, three young classical violinists – Aaliya, Nisha and Naima Ramakrishnan – play a few of the lighter pieces from the Western canon. The children, some of whom are heartbreakingly thin and bald under their Santa hats, listen patiently but when the duo break into the popular dance number 'Zingaat' from the Marathi film *Sairat*, the delight of the familiar floods their faces.

An Interdisciplinary Approach to Healthcare

I come back to do a round with Monica Santos, clown and social entrepreneur. She is magical with the children of course, but when she walks into the ward, everyone starts smiling: the nurses and ward boys, the ayahs and the parents. The atmosphere shifts and lightens for a little while at least.

Santos, a Spanish national who has been in India for years, was into theatre when the discovery of clowning changed her life. 'I discovered that you use your vulnerabilities, you use your miseries, and you make people laugh, and that is super-cathartic. But more than laughter, I can be there for the patient,' she says.

Santos tells me, 'I know my job looks like "silliness and stupidity", but I take it seriously. I am a professional. This is my work and so I maintain meticulous reports about everything.'

When she checks in for her day at Wadia Hospital, she first checks in with the palliative care unit and gets updates. 'One of the nurses or social workers tells me what's happening. I get not only the medical information but the social history of the patient as well. It makes me a better clown, a more situation-specific clown. If I am told that there has been a disagreement between the parents, I can work on easing the situation. And when I come back to the unit, I debrief too because as a clown I see things others will not – I see what the child is going through.'

The benefits to the children from books, music, dancing and laughter are many. They report decreased pain, family communication is enhanced, and they say they now have more friends in the ward. They have all had a reason to smile in these sessions and when the activity is over, they can talk about the moments of fun and smile again.

The hospital's homecare palliative services began in 2022; the team does more than sixty homecare visits every month, mostly for children with chronic illnesses, like cerebral palsy.

Dr Lakshmi Krishnan, the homecare physician, explains, 'There are cases where the parents have to tube feed the child. When we go for these visits, we assess the family's resources – material, human and social. Who is at home? Who cares for the child? Are there relatives close at hand? Do the neighbours pitch in? End-of-life patients become high priority. We work to manage pain, improve the quality of life, and provide emotional support to the child and the family.'

It's not just the varied team roles but also the commitment to empathetic patient-centred care that stands out at Wadia Hospital. I realize this when on one visit I attend a workshop on washing the bodies of babies who have just died. I cannot say I thought this would be the high point of my week but there was something very uplifting and humbling about it in the end. The small frame that had faced life for so short a period, the faces gathered around made solemn by this dread burden. It was as if each one of us were being asked: You who have lived so long, you who were given this life, what use have you made of it?

I speak with Anuradha Karegar, consultant psychologist, who explains the rationale behind the workshop. 'Dr Veronique believes we must all, every one of us who works here at Wadia, be trained in palliative care. We want the maushis to treat those bodies with respect and gentleness. We also work with our security staff. Families can become violent when a child dies and attack the doctors, but we all know where that anger is coming from. And it can be minimized, contained, if you have worked with people so that they treat this mixture of grief and rage with care and concern.'

Now doctors from the maternity and neonatology wards of Nowrojee Wadia Hospital, which stands across the road from the children's hospital, have begun contacting the palliative care unit at Wadia Children's Hospital. The palliative care team walks over when a child is likely to be born with complications so severe that they may not live very long outside the sterile environment of incubators and life-support machines.

Karegar says, 'It takes some doing. But hard as this is, we now have a plan. The baby is given to the mother. The father gets a chance to hold the baby too. They weep, they nuzzle it, they hold it as if it were the most precious thing in the world. They blow at their baby sometimes or pray over the little thing or wet their baby's lips with holy water. This contact with life is fleeting but it is also intense. And in some way, they begin the process of dealing with the death of their child even in the last few moments of that short life.'

She pauses a moment to add, 'I wonder why all hospitals that have an obstetrics and gynaecology department don't have palliative care units. This is not just about the health of mothers and babies, this is also about the future of the human race.'

I walked into the ward and a young man walks in. He has had a cancer relapse and is back for a second round of chemotherapy, but he says he is still attending college. Karegar asks if he is taking care. He says he wears a mask on the bus to college and carries his own food and water.

'Sometimes people ask, "What is the point of them taking an exam if they have only a few months to live?" And that's not the right question because you're not living their lives. Often young men with terminal illnesses will want to drive a vehicle once in their lives, and we always say, "Yes, you should, but get your driving licence first." And then comes the question of why waste time on a driving licence. The answer is simple,' Karegar says. 'It is not your time here; it is his time and he should get to do what he wants with it.'

5

Comfort, Where You Are

'I was born in this bed,' my maternal grandmother, Bertha Tellis nee Pinto, said to me, pointing to a four-poster in Porvorim, Goa. We were standing in her ancestral home on one of my rare visits as a young man to my home state. 'My mother nursed all her six children here. My elder sister died of influenza in this bed. My mother suffered through her last illness in this bed. And when she died, she was laid out in this bed too.'

That bed was the locus of many medical histories in my family. But this was in the days before hospitals became the only place where care could be accessed. These days, medical help does not come to you; you go looking for it. Here again, palliative care differs from the practice of medicine. It shows up where you need it the most. There are three spaces where palliative care is generally to be found – at a hospital, at the patient's home and at a palliative care centre.

Hospital-based Palliative Care

Dr Nandini Vallath at St John's Hospital, Bengaluru, remembers when she first started her practice as an anaesthesiologist: 'A patient with cancer pain came to me. I was doing nerve blocks at the time. I found the nerve; I blocked it, and the patient did experience relief from the pain. But then I heard that he had committed suicide. That shook me. Looking back, I can see that I had not talked to the patient as a person, not seen his depression, not asked after him as a human being, not even considered him one. I had not done my due diligence, but then that was because I did not know there was a due diligence to do. I wish I had a palliative care team within the hospital that could have supported me to see the patient beyond the illness.'

It would seem natural that patients should first receive palliative care when they are under the care of their treating physician at a hospital either admitted as an inpatient or visiting an OPD.

It will be a while before this becomes the norm across the country. But in hospitals where palliative care is being made available, it's heartening to see treating physicians and palliative care professionals finding ways to come together to hold patients and families in a reassuring circle of care.

Dr Ira Almeida explains that since they started palliative care at South Goa District Hospital, the treating physicians have been introduced to a 'checklist' that alerts them to call in the palliative team. 'This is a simple checklist that assesses the functional status of the patient, the presence of comorbidities and the emotional condition of the patient and caregiver. The treating physician knows that a score higher than 4 means they should refer to the palliative care team.'

At times, however, in busy hospitals, physicians are unable to make a connection with the palliative care team. In such overburdened facilities, the palliative care team members will also often fan out through the inpatient department and watch for signs of distress. Sometimes a nurse might report a weeping caregiver or a confused patient. Once the team has been alerted, it checks with the treating physician, and then the palliative care doctor will meet with the patient and caregiver and tell them about palliative care services.

A needs assessment survey is then conducted to understand the situation in which the patient finds herself or himself. This includes not just details of the disease and the symptoms but also the family situation, whether the patient is likely to find a supportive environment at home, the economic situation, the kind of work the patient does, whether this will be made difficult over time, and the distress the patient feels. Distress is now being seen as the sixth vital sign that is as important as pulse or temperature.

'The first encounter,' says Lalita Bhavani, social worker with PRPCS, Hyderabad, 'is like detective work. You have to listen hard and pick up clues. A patient generally does not open up immediately. Trust grows slowly because the encounter is often staged in the middle of a noisy hospital ward, not under ideal conditions. But when you keep coming back and you're still there and they see you mean well, they begin to tell you their worries. Sometimes it is about the food, sometimes about the rent, but I have learned that there is nothing off topic. If you are fully there for the patient, they begin to see it and open up. It takes time, but in palliative care, you must give them the sense that you have all the time in the world for them.'

The OPD in a hospital may also be, in many cases, the site of the first encounter. These may be brief, but the hope is that the information and perspective provided by the team at the palliative care OPD will form a bond of trust so that the patient and the caregiver know that they are not alone.

The Cipla Palliative Care Centre supports palliative care OPDs in government and charitable hospitals in Pune. Dr Sonali Kulkarni, who leads this work, says: 'At the government hospital, our social worker and clinical psychologist sit in the same OPD as the oncologist, so the patient and caregiver see the palliative care team as an extension of the treatment support. In the charitable hospital we work in, we have a separate OPD. The oncologists now just have to say, 'Go to OPD 23', and we speak with patients and their families, assess their needs and link them to the necessary support. We have daily updates to the oncologists on our interventions so that together we form a network of care for that patient and caregiver.'

The palliative care team addressing the needs of inpatients or OPD patients will have many roles to play; they will often form a bridge between the medical system and the patient. They will seek answers to questions the patients might have and reinforce the importance of following medical protocols. They will also help them navigate through the complex systems of the hospital and they will be on hand to answer questions and confront fears and doubts.

But eventually, those with life-limiting or chronic diseases must go home – indeed, they often long to go home. And so, home visits by palliative care teams are available for them too.

Home-based Palliative Care

When I visited Homi Bhabha Cancer Hospital and Research Centre at Visakhapatnam, I spent the morning getting to know the team and then we set off on home visits.

The first home visit clarifies what it means to be poor and ill in a village in India. M. Janakiamma is somewhere between fifty-five and sixty years old. She was in end-of-life care when she was put on oral chemotherapy and responded very well. Her lung cancer had her nearly bedridden but now she even does some cooking. It is a baking hot May afternoon and when we arrive, only her husband is present.

Janakiamma has gone to cool off a little with a friend down the road. As she limps back home, halfway down the road, Dr Tejeshwar Rao, the palliative care physician, reaches out to help. She shrugs him off as if to say, 'I've got this.'

Her independence is astonishing, but when I hear her story, I see its roots. Janakiamma and her husband are alone in the world. They get by on a pension of Rs 2,500 and the kindness of the community. Their home is tiny, and they cook on a wood fire, which cannot be doing her lungs any good.

We sit on the ground where Janakiamma is comfortable. This is in keeping with Dr Cicley Saunders's instructions to all the doctors who worked with her. They were not to loom over the patient but sit down by the bedside. This not only suggests equality since the doctor and patient would be on eye level but also suggests that the doctor has time for the patient, and that this is no rushed, impersonal 'doctor's visit'.

Janakiamma's blood pressure is taken and her medications are looked over. The social worker is quietly topping up the dry rations, also part of the service. Janakiamma's husband hovers around, protective, interested. He proffers a booklet which the doctor checks over and updates. Each home has some variant of this booklet. In some cases, it is a file, and in others, a notebook that contains all the details, the social, medical and psychological history of the patient, the medications they are taking and all the other relevant details. This document helps the doctor or health professional locate the patient on the spectrum of palliative care.

All seems to be well, and after some civilities, we set out again.

Over the next few months, I see this scenario play out in various forms and spaces across the country. There is a visit to a high-rise where a retired police officer brings out bloodstained rags from the night before. There is a stopover at a small hut tucked away behind a university campus where a young man hurriedly extinguishes his beedi when he sees us coming. There's a halt at a home where several dogs emerge from under the bed of a near-comatose woman. They are subdued but they will not leave her side.

Comfort, Where You Are

My abiding memory of these visits is that of a car and a driver and a nurse and a doctor and a mental health professional bumping along country roads, looking for someone's home, and of a general welcome once we arrive. But then who would not welcome the palliative care team? A doctor who comes to you where you are? With a nurse and a counsellor in tow? Perhaps carrying a stash of your medications? Rolls of bandage and fresh adult diapers? Sometimes even carrying dry rations?

'At times we face slammed doors,' Dr Samina Mohamed, medical officer at PRPCS. 'Sometimes people are afraid of the stigma of ill health. They do not want it to be known that there is something in their homes that they cannot deal with on their own. So, they may even agree to allow us to visit them, but then, when we come all the way, the door is locked and they do not answer calls.'

However, once the breakthrough is made and the door is opened, things change dramatically. On the dozens of home visits to which I have been a silent witness across the country, from Guwahati to Delhi to Hyderabad, from Bengaluru to Mumbai to Thiruvananthapuram, the palliative care team was always welcome. We were always offered tea, and sometimes fizzy cold drinks manifested. The little ones put on their best clothes and preened and were fussed over by the nurses.

When asked if home care tends to be more expensive than hospital-based care, Dr Jayarajan Ponissery of the Cipla Palliative Care Centre, Pune, says: 'Home care may require greater coordination, human resource efforts and investment than hospital care, but these things cannot be compared without looking at the context. Consider catheterization. Say the patient can no longer pass urine and needs a catheter inserted. With home care, the catheter comes to them with a nurse adept at doing this who has time to do it. If the patient is to go to a hospital, then a caregiver must take a day's leave. This is a cost. Then there is the cost of transportation. If you are going to a private hospital, the procedure will involve a cost. If you are going to a government hospital, you are faced with an interminable wait and the psychological cost of being treated by some overworked person who may, out of fatigue, lash out at you. By contrast, when the care comes to you, you are in your own home. You are king there. You are in control.'

Comfort, Where You Are

At the Indian Association for Palliative Care Conference, 2024, Dr M.T. Bhatia, who started the Palliative Care Centre at the Gujarat Cancer & Research Institute, also disagrees when he is told that home care is seen as expensive. 'In an ICU you are separated from your family when you need them the most, you are prodded and poked by strangers, you are woken up at 4 a.m. for some procedure. Much of what is done in hospitals can be done at home. We can train the caregivers to do what needs to be done and to identify emergencies. Home is where the patient will be treated with love and care, and that is what every human being needs.'

What Dr Bhatia says about the family being able to learn to do much of the work of the hospital is proved to me on a visit to Sangam Vihar, a dense tenement sprawl in Delhi, with the CanSupport team. Irfan is a petty trader with a small shop that he manages. He has been shifted to palliative care since his oral cancer metastasized and left two open wounds in his cheek.

When the door is opened, we are told that Irfan has gone to the shop. He works there for a few hours every day. A child is sent scuttling off to fetch her father, while we step in and meet his wife.

Irfan returns at this point. His face is swathed in a handkerchief; it looks as if he is masked up as part of the COVID-19 prevention protocol. I brace as he pulls down the handkerchief, but though I can see his teeth through his cheek, the wounds are clean and have no discernible smell and the skin is pink in places. The wounds have been tended well. His wife must be proud of her handiwork.

'When these close up,' Irfan says. 'I will have no trouble.'

'Are you having trouble now?' Dr Sanjay Sharma asks. Dr Sharma turned to palliative care after decades of work in a corporate hospital. A nurse who knew him in the hospital setting had joined CanSupport and she urged him to come and see the kind of work they did. He came for a day, and the next day, he handed in his resignation at the hospital. He had found his métier.

Irfan explains his problems: 'My friends say COVID-19 is over and they try and pull off my mask.'

It is obvious that Irfan has kept his condition a secret from his friends. But this has turned him into something of a social recluse.

'It will take him some time to realize that there are things he can no longer do,' says Dr Sharma later.

He steps in for a quiet conversation with Irfan. Irfan does much of the talking, and the doctor nods and listens. There are times when he stops nodding.

We step out into the sun.

Dr Sanjay Sharma sighs. Something has shaken him, despite all his experience with illness and pain.

'These stories change you,' he says. 'They change you as a doctor and as a person.'

The Palliative Care Centre

For many, perhaps home is the best place to receive care. But what if home is a shelter under a flyover? What if home is already stretched to its limits in terms of caring for bedridden and old people and the potential caregivers must work? That's when palliative care centres can be a blessing.

A palliative care centre is sometimes also called a hospice, though the two are not the same. Unlike a hospice, which focuses on end-of-life care in a sense, helping one die with minimum pain and distress, the focus in a palliative care centre is on quality of life and on pain and symptom management at any stage of an illness, whether terminal or not.

Like many people, I did not make the distinction, and I was somewhat apprehensive on the day I visited my first palliative care unit, expecting it to be about death and dying. But the Cipla Palliative Care Centre in Warje, Pune, turned out to be completely different from my expectations.

It was about life, and the joy and comfort that can be derived from life for as long as we have it. The wards, flooded with natural light, opened out to beautiful gardens and were named after the flowers that grew outside. The beds were filled with patients attending to their phones, reading or sleeping. Where a hospital sometimes feels frantic, the Cipla centre was rich in serenity and acceptance. And there was a sense of being in a large yet intimate home. I saw the patients being referred to by their names and not by their bed number. It was a place of life as patients saw others go home with their pain was so well managed that they were looking forward to celebrating festivals and birthdays again.

'We do not say "They have come here to die",' said Dr Vivek Nirabhawane, previously head of clinical services at the centre. 'We say that they have come here to live their days to the fullest.'

When I see Holi (the festival of colours) being celebrated at the centre, I know what he means. The sight of patients, their faces with colours and smiles, filled the space with a rare kind of hope. In those moments, it wasn't about the pain or the prognosis – it was about the joy of being present, celebrating life in all its vivid shades. For a while, the air was thick with love and togetherness, momentarily blurring the lines between patient and caregiver, illness and wellness.

I found the same sense of peace and calm when I stepped into Karunashraya in Bengaluru. I was struck by how different it felt from the typical sterile, hospital-like atmosphere. The design here is open and inviting, with lush gardens, breezy courtyards and calming water bodies scattered throughout. Sunlight streams into the wards, filling hope and beauty into life's most challenging times – it is architecture with heart, a space that feels healing not just physically but also emotionally.

I am told of how Laila, a lady of some years and much living, wanted a tattoo to mark the seven years that she had been free of the cancer that had returned now. The Karunashraya team had to battle the lockdown to find a tattoo artist, but he was located. He came to the centre and gave Laila her tattoo. A month later, she was buried in the red dress of her own choosing.

The problem in India is that most people with chronic or life-limiting diseases end their days in the worst possible environment: the ICU.

Dr Priya Thomas, who heads the palliative care unit at NIMHANS, Bengaluru, says: 'Key to managing an end-of-life situation is advance care planning. But people are not ready to talk about death. We are a country that believes deeply in magic and lives in the hope of miracles. The families of patients will say to a doctor, "Yes, the textbooks say that this is incurable, but anything is possible, no, doctor?" They will tell you how someone's friend's cousin recovered and lived for ten years when the doctors gave him two months. Finally, the doctor will say, "Yes, I suppose anything can happen," and the family hears this as "Yes, a miracle is on its way."'

Sometimes a miracle does materialize, but more often than not the patient ends up on a ventilator. Dr Thomas adds, 'With ventilators in corporate hospitals, it is often the family's financial constraints that will decide when it is turned off. This is all closely linked to our concepts of relationships and regrets. We have no system for talking about difficult matters. Because we never talk about death. Death is inevitable, the only inevitable thing if you have been born. But few of us plan for it and know how to deal with it. Death can break a family.'

And the saddest part of this is how that death happens when it comes in the ICU: away from loved ones, away from familiar sounds and touch, poked and prodded by young doctors – good, well-meaning people but too eager to learn how to perform medical interventions. Alone, isolated and bewildered – this is no way for a human being to die.

Palliative care thus seeks to place the patient at the centre of a care collective. A patient is seen as a human being and not as a condition or a disease. For most people, this circle of caring is the family, but sometimes specialized care and round-the-clock nursing is needed, and then patients are advised to seek palliative care in a hospital setting. This need does not always signal that the end is near.

As I walk around with Dr Leena Gangoli at Sukoon Nilaya, Mumbai's first inclusive palliative care inpatient centre, I meet Mala, fifty-five years old and grappling with anaemia, diabetes, hypertension and the aftermath of two strokes. Her husband died last year, and she finds herself dependent on her son Raju for daily care. Her other sons have distanced themselves, unable to cope with her deteriorating health. Raju, dedicated but overwhelmed, has quit his job to attend to his mother's needs, and their relationship is strained, reflecting the challenges they faced.

The Sukoon Nilaya team recognized that Mala's path to recovery required addressing not only her physical symptoms but also her emotional and social well-being. Despite initial discouragement and resistance, they persisted in their efforts to engage both mother and son in a supportive environment at the centre. The team managed her fatigue through diet and exercise, and helped her regain the use of her hands with physiotherapy to get her more independent. When the social worker spoke to Mala, she mentioned that she was depressed because of her loss of vision. Through Sukoon Nilaya's network, she was referred to a community camp, where she received her much-needed eye surgery and ongoing care at no cost. This intervention proved transformative, as restored vision not only enhanced her daily activities but also revitalized her participation in rehabilitation.

With improved sight came renewed hope, Mala began mobility training at Sukoon Nilaya, a step-by-step process that gradually restored her ability to walk independently.

Mala's journey is a testament to the power of integrated palliative care. Through careful coordination and compassionate support, her journey from dependency to regained mobility and improved vision exemplifies the profound impact of community outreach and family dedication in holistic healthcare.

Studies have shown that palliative care can actually increase life expectancy. This makes sense, in a way. The patient is well cared for, fed properly, given physiotherapy and occupational therapy, settled into a stable routine, all of which points to an improvement in general health.

'We had a family come to us and say that they had been advised by the hospital to take their father home,' a CanSupport counsellor in Delhi told me. 'They were told, "*Woh do dinon ka mehmaan hai*" (He has only a couple of days left to live). Perhaps whoever had said this to them meant it as a metaphor, but the family took this literally. First, we had to tell them that no one can predict death accurately. But when we had got past all that, worked with them, and created a plan for his care, he lived a life on his own terms for six more months. His family had a chance to say goodbye, to prepare and to rest easier knowing that he was pain-free in those last months.'

Many physicians, however, think of a palliative care centre as the solution only when the home situation does not allow for care. But patients who can come to palliative care centres can also get to go home for short breaks or special events. 'Patients can get tired of the routine from time to time,' says Dr Babita Varkey at Karunashraya. 'Then they say they want to go home. They spend some time there and then perhaps they remember what they have here and then they come back of their own accord. Patient autonomy is the key.'

Palliative care teams spend a lot of time listening – listening primarily to the patient, but also to the caregivers and decision-makers. But the mandate of the palliative care team is to make sure the patient – so often reduced to a disease, so often made invisible by gown and mask and hairnet, so often ignored in conversation – is returned to the status of a human being. It is their job to consider the patient in time. Who the patient was before the disease is as important as what the patient is experiencing in the present; the team must also bear in mind what the patient is likely to experience in the future.

But it is also the palliative care team's job to consider the patient in the family, society and the larger world. It is their job to know what the patient wants from the present and from the future. This is often easier to do in a palliative care centre.

———

I think of a moment when I was sitting with Dr Philomena D'Souza at Novi Survat, the palliative care centre for children in Porvorim, Goa. A woman walked past us into the facility with her nine-year-old daughter draped over a shoulder as one might carry a towel.

'Yes,' she said, looking at my open mouth and slack jaw. 'Yes. We send our vehicle to pick up the children who come here for therapy but this is the last mile. Each parent has their own way of carrying the child.'

She stops to think.

'Novi Survat opens its arms to all children. There are those struggling with cancer or a relapse but there are also those who have Down syndrome, muscular dystrophy, congenital disorders, those with non-standard organs. What do we do about these children of ours? They are often in and out of hospitals, which means that education gets disrupted, development is staggered. If there is no timely and regular intervention, the child's physical, mental and emotional development can stop. It can even regress. You want to ask the parents: Why didn't you bring them? Why are you skipping sessions? Then you see what they are up against, these doughty women who are fighting to keep their heads above water. You see the enormity of the problem and equally you feel the helplessness of your situation. But then the child smiles at you and demonstrates proudly something they have just learned, something they couldn't do yesterday and then the world shrinks to that moment. You know then that you are called on to do what you can with that child and their parents, to forget everything else. You must aim high. You must aim at the best possible treatment for this child and this family. This is idealistic but if you lower your standards, you will give what you can give rather than what you should give.'

Give what you should, not what you can. That sounds great. But how will you know what you should give?

Dr Ira Almeida has an answer: 'If only we could get this "they-should-be-grateful" lens out of our eyes and change it to the "how-would-I-like-to-be-treated" lens, things would change suddenly and dramatically. Patients might be seen as people. They might be brought into a circle of caring. They might be freed from the burden of gratitude and allow themselves the pleasure of having expectations from the health systems built to serve them.'

6

Listening and Sharing

Dr Rajam Iyer, a cheerful pulmonologist and now a palliative care specialist who practices at both P.D. Hinduja National Hospital and Medical Research Centre and Bhatia Hospital in Mumbai, has had some personal experiences with palliative care that taught her the value of communication. The down-to-earth Dr Iyer became a pulmonologist in 1995. In 2002, she went to England to get her Membership of the Royal Colleges of Physicians of the United Kingdom (MRCP [UK]), and in 2010 she was back in Mumbai and began to work with Dr Sujeet Rajan, a pulmonologist with over twenty-five years of experience.

Reflecting on a deeply personal moment, Dr Iyer shares, 'In 2015, I lost my dad. He had a stroke, and after the MRI the doctors said, "We won't be doing much for him," so I said to myself, "I can do this at home." I took him home, and almost immediately he began dipping in and out of consciousness. So, we kept him clean and generally comfortable. He lived on for three weeks with all of us around him praying, laughing, singing, crying.'

She pauses now to think about this, but back then there must not have been much time to process the grief around her father's death as the family soon faced another medical crisis.

'Barely fourteen days after my father's passing, my mother came down with pneumonia. I had her admitted to the ICU. There, she asked me, "You didn't take your father to hospital. Why did you take me?" I said, "His illness was irreversible. What you have is pneumonia, and that can be treated. When a disease is reversible, I will do everything in my power." My mother looked at me intently and said, "If something irreversible happens to me, I want no hospital, no ICU." I agreed.'

She sighs. 'In India, communication is very poor. We are taught that patient autonomy is the first principle of medical ethics, and yet we don't always ask the patient what they want. I didn't ask my father how he wanted to be cared for in the end and probably wouldn't have known my mother's wishes if she hadn't categorically spelled them out for me.'

Something about all this made Dr Iyer feel she should re-examine her clinical practice.

'In 2016, I took myself to Pallium India in Thiruvananthapuram. In 2017, I did a fellowship in Calicut and in 2018, a palliative care diploma from Cardiff. Back then, I did not identify what I did for my father – keeping him comfortable at home instead of being hooked to a ventilator – as palliative care; I just acted on instinct. My only regret is that I did not discuss this with him. But it allowed me and my mother to discuss her wishes.'

Sometime later that day, I attend a Continuing Medical Education (CME) seminar in a huge hall at Hinduja Hospital, Mumbai, where Dr Iyer asks a loaded question: 'How many of you are comfortable talking about death with your patients?'

There are about a hundred doctors in the room and only one hand went up, pointing to a real need for more difficult conversations in healthcare.

Why Communication Matters

Communication is not just the life breath of palliative care, it also underlies the whole of medicine. Your body talks to itself all the time. When you cough or sneeze, that's one part of the body telling another to expel an irritant. When you feel an itch, that's your body signalling the need to deal with a skin situation. And when your body talks to you in the form of pain, distress or unease, that's your nervous system telling you that something is wrong.

You then communicate this to your doctor, who must listen to you and decide what to do about it. Perhaps the doctor takes your temperature – that's your body talking, communication mediated through a machine. Next, the doctor orders a battery of tests, and your body will now speak in the language of numbers. The doctor sorts through a personal database of information and experience and makes a diagnosis. This must now be communicated to you, and in many cases, it is as simple as taking your meds on time, adjusting your diet, taking some exercise and getting enough sleep.

In an increasingly competitive world, where specializations and super-specializations are much sought after, the general practitioner – the family physician in their little clinic, filled with patients who know each other – is under threat. Now, one might visit a clinic and meet doctors who only know what you tell them. The emphasis in this environment has been shifted to being a good diagnostician and being up to date with the pharmacological armoury. Communication? How can that be of any importance between two complete strangers who may never see each other again?

The worst moments come after diagnosis, says Ms Poonam Bagai, a cancer survivor and founder of CanKids KidsCan,* an NGO in New Delhi that offers comprehensive care to children with cancer. 'In a large hospital with so many patients, doctors might deliver difficult news, like a cancer diagnosis, and quickly move on to the next. The family is left in shock, without the support they need to process the information. There's no one to sit with them, offer comfort or listen to their story – how they've been struggling, what steps they've already taken and how they arrived at this point. Without emotional support,

---

*They are popularly known as CanKids.

it's much harder for families to absorb the news or figure out what comes next.'

It is at this point that the palliative care team must come in to ease the stress of the moment. Dr Poonam Wade, Professor (Addl.), Department of Paediatrics, TN Medical College and BYL Nair Municipal Hospital, Mumbai, says, 'Families facing serious illness often need explanations multiple times to truly understand the issues. This can be tough in busy hospitals like ours where doctors see hundreds of patients daily. The lack of emotional support in such situations can lead to tremendous stress, feelings of fear, helplessness, frustration and uncertainty. A good palliative care team can step in to ease the doctor's burden. We need dedicated doctors, psychologists and social workers to have open and honest communication tailored to each family's needs, and to create access to support groups and resources.'

At Karunashraya, Michelle Normen, who heads a team of six counsellors, tells me how good communication can help patients stick to their treatment routines and so improve their chances. She was working at the Adyar Cancer Institute, Chennai, where it was found that patients did not adhere to the drugs protocol for a condition known as non-adherent chronic myeloid leukaemia, which caused fatigue and led to infections, anaemia and bleeding.

The treatment was free. It did not cure the patient but it turned the disease into something that could be managed, like diabetes.

And yet, one-third of the patients would simply stop. Many of the patients from the low socio-economic status groups did not even know what the disease was about. Some would not tell their family. A patient got married without telling her husband about her condition. What troubled them the most, though, was that each time they came, they would find another doctor there. There was no feeling of continuity. They were reluctant to share the side effects like hyperpigmentation or itching. After all, they felt they were being treated for leukaemia, how could they complain about dark spots?

'We also found that they were not taking their medications according to the prescriptions because of lack of information. There was hardly any conversation between the doctor and the patient. And so, we established a new protocol. After diagnosis, they would be taken to a room to see a video that explained what the disease was and how they should take their medications. After that they would talk to the social worker. We also started monitoring for side effects.'

Adherence improved, says Michelle, because there was someone to talk to, to clear up questions about having children and such. But most of all it was because they had someone to reach out to with questions.

There are also tangible economic benefits to good communication, points out Dr Naveen Salins, professor at and head of the Department of Palliative Medicine at Kasturba Medical College, Manipal. He says, 'When I was in Australia, we had to buy indemnity insurance – in case someone sues you, if you had communication training, your premiums were lower. Because studies have shown that 75 per cent of malpractice cases are because of poor communication. Only 25 per cent are because of errors. And in that 25 per cent, if the doctor is honest, it goes down to 5 per cent. If the doctor says, "I am very sorry that this happened. I made a mistake", most of the times it is accepted.'

He adds, 'Attacks on doctors are caused partly by poor communication skills and bad management of expectations, and these are linked. A lot of communication skills are non-verbal too: making patients feel valued and respected.'

Communication is vital and especially so with children, who are almost always kept out of the loop. Professor Julia Downing, chief executive of the International Children's Palliative Care Network (ICPCN), is an experienced palliative care nurse, educationalist and researcher with a PhD in palliative care education. At the conference of the IAPC in 2024, she told the audience a story:

'Children who have been ill for a while have had the time to think about life and death. If they are in a ward for a while, they have seen children come and go, and some of those children have died. Among them, there may have been friends. I remember a twelve-year-old girl, whose friend died one night. The next morning, the twelve-year-old was asking everyone – the nurses, the doctors on the rounds, the cleaners, everyone – what had happened to the child. We met her later in the day and when we told her that the child had died, she said that she had known this all along.

"'So why were you asking?'

"'I just wanted to find out who would tell me the truth when my turn comes."

'There was silence in the room as many of the doctors there tried to absorb the maturity of this child.'

Good Communication Can Be Taught

I am reminded of a Continuing Medical Education seminar I attended at Delhi's AIIMS. I was invited to speak on the problem of caregiving in the context of mental illness based on my experience of it, which I had used in the novel *Em and the Big Hoom* and in the collection of caregiver accounts I had edited, *A Book of Light: When a Loved One Has a Different Mind*. At the plenary, a renowned nephrologist told us about his experience of a very early, difficult conversation with one of his patients. He told the patient he had irreversible kidney failure in so many words – plainly, flatly. The patient's wife followed him out of the room and told him in no uncertain terms that for all his education and degrees, he was not a doctor. He was not a healer, she said, because he had no idea how to talk to a patient.

It took me back to my conversation with Dr Naveen Salins: 'We did a project recently on communication with the emergency medicine department. Eighty students were in the project. We got an actor, who was given a script, and an independent psychologist to assess the students; the psychologist was given a checklist. We would do an intervention and then repeat the experiment. We found that communication was a learned skill. You get better at it as you do it.'

In my own experience of thirty-five years as a teacher, I have found that the best incentive for students is marks. The pass–fail binary is what keeps students going. Dr Salins agrees: 'I have been an examiner on foreign exams. There are stations they have to pass. Communication is one of those stations. Even if they pass the other stations and fail communication, they fail the exams.'

As a result of nearly twenty years of work, led by Pallium India, in 2010, palliative care was included in the curriculum of the MBBS degree. When I set out to write this book, most of the senior doctors I interviewed said that they had gone through all of medical college and even specializations without even hearing the term palliative care. That is slowly changing since Attitude, Ethics, and Communication Skills (AETCOM) became a part of the syllabus in 2019 and includes 144 hours of training. Forty of these hours are devoted to communication.

But the problem may also lie with how communication is taught at medical colleges in India. Dr Jayita Deodhar, professor at and head of the Department of Palliative Medicine, TMH, Mumbai, says, 'Medical education in India often focuses heavily on didactic teaching and theoretical concepts, leaving little room for practical communication training like role plays. The pressure to prioritize diagnostic and management skills, combined with understaffed and overburdened healthcare systems, means communication training often gets overlooked in our medical colleges.'

She adds, 'To fix this, we need to make serious investments in healthcare and train all staff to communicate effectively. From day one, medical education should highlight the importance of these skills. A well-structured curriculum that includes both theory and practical exercises like role plays is key. Technology, skills labs, and partnerships with patients, patient groups and even actors can help create a more hands-on and engaging way to teach communication. This way, we can ensure that good communication becomes second nature for healthcare professionals.'

Getting communication right, however, is not rocket science. It is about empathy. You simply ask yourself: How would I like to be treated in the same situation? Would you like to be eye-to-eye with your doctor or would you rather the doctor loomed over you and told you what was going on from on high? By the same token, perhaps it is best not to respond to cell phone calls – or at least to explain how important they are before answering them. Instructions must be given to other staff not to disturb the conversation unless it is an emergency.

Dr Suchi Gaonkar of the Goa Medical College and Hospital says: 'When I am with a patient, I try to be there fully. I try to focus on what they are telling me. There are some things they tell me about to which I can find solutions and then I must be solution driven. There are other things they tell me that they simply want to say out loud. They want to be heard. They want you to listen. Then I must be simply a hundred per cent in the moment and with them. To decide which are the ones that need solutions and which are the ones that just need to be listened to can take a lot of energy, but that is the job.'

Talking Through Tough Times

Sometimes a doctor must have a very difficult conversation with a patient diagnosed with a serious illness such as dementia or congestive heart failure. The difficulty lies in the patient's reaction. The uncertainty is over but the diagnosis brings its own share of trauma. The pain has just become suffering.

Dr Rajam Iyer puts it well: 'Nobody budgets for suffering. And yet it is universal in a hospital. Everyone who comes here carries some suffering with them.'

Dr Roop Gursahani, neurologist at Hinduja Hospital, Mumbai, says, 'A diagnosis of any serious illness is akin to dropping a bomb on your patient's life. Everything changes from that moment. They need time to understand it and they need your attention.'

Communication is not just about how one speaks but also about who speaks, to whom, and how. Dr Nandini Vallath of St John's Hospital discovered this when she was working in palliative care at a corporate hospital. 'On rounds one day, a well-educated and well-to-do patient said to me: "I'm tired. I don't want any more curative treatments." So, I went and told his doctor that. The doctor said: "Dr Nandini, your job is to deal with his pain. Leave us to do the rest." I learned a lesson from that. When the patient said it to me again the next week, I told him: "You have to tell your doctor this." Then I equipped him with some ways to say it. I ran through some scenarios: what his doctor might say and how he was to respond. That rehearsal helped him; he was allowed to go home – he was freed from what he had begun to see as an onslaught.'

Palliative care is also about empowering the patient to face down the system. Dr Vallath says, 'I think we should always ask what the goals of treatment are, not set them ourselves. That is how we respect the person we are treating.'

Dr Sujeet Rajan is a renowned Mumbai-based pulmonologist with Bhatia Hospital and Bombay Hospital who has managed to get palliative care into the latter, which is a private hospital. He says: 'We have it all right now. We have all the drugs, we have the best prices, we have chemists everywhere. Now we need to work on doctors' communication skills. I talked to a young doctor at AIIMS. He said, "We are being taught communication. But we are being told what to communicate rather than how to communicate. And that's wrong."'

'Palliative care is about nuance,' Dr Rajan continues. 'It is about things said but as much about things left unsaid. Nuance is not about preaching. These are things that cannot be taught because you learn them on the job, you learn them out of failures, you learn them from small successes when you manage to make a change for the patient and the caregiver, and that change is for the better. You store that away, but you cannot use it as it is. You will need to work it out again for the next patient. But there are still some basic things that you learn which will always be useful.'

The more time health professionals spend with their patients, the more they listen and the more they learn.

Sheila Cassidy is a British physician who went to Chile in the early 1970s where, after treating a wounded revolutionary, she was arrested, imprisoned and tortured. When she returned to England, she became the director of a small hospice. In her book, *Sharing the Darkness: The Spirituality of Caring* (1991), she writes: 'Perhaps all nurses and doctors should "role play" being a patient every couple of years. They should learn what it feels like to be wheeled down the corridor on a stretcher in a paper hat, to have the various "routine" investigations, they should know that having blood tests is sometimes very painful, and that having metal instruments inserted into various bodily orifices can be very unpleasant indeed. More than anything, they should remember how horrid it is to feel foolish or misunderstood and that the fear of being thought neurotic is often worse than the finding of a genuine pathology!'

One might say that a difficult conversation is also a necessary conversation. And if it is difficult for the patient, it is difficult for the doctor too. Dr Sujeet Rajan says, 'I can't have more than a couple of those conversations every day. I don't think it is possible to take on more than that and still be present, responsive and understanding. I try to schedule them for the morning because many of my patients are older people and will have sleepless nights if they are told of this late in the evening.'

Techniques can be learned; caring must be innate. And when technique falters, caring works wonders.

As Dr Anitha Haribalakrishna, associate professor and head of the Department of Neonatology at King Edward Memorial Hospital, Mumbai, which leads a neonatal palliative care programme at the hospital, says, 'While perfect medical techniques are essential, empathy and care humanize healthcare, making it more relatable and personal. By combining technical expertise with compassion, healthcare providers can deliver more comprehensive and effective care. Empathy is essential for holistic healing. By managing expectations and providing realistic hope, effective communication can mitigate imperfections in treatment. Ultimately, it promotes collaboration, trust and better health outcomes, even when treatment is not perfect.'

'Why Me?'

'Why me?' is a question that has occurred to all of us at some point. I must have asked it of myself a thousand times. Once I must have even asked it aloud in the presence of my friend, the sociologist and thinker Rudolf Heredia, who said, 'It is a question that never arises when something good happens to you.

We all feel we merit the good things that happen to us, they are the logical outcome of our goodness. It is the bad things that surprise the question out of us.'

I remember being angry at the lack of empathy, startled at the severity and elegance of the logic of this. I also made a note that it was not the kind of answer you could give someone who was really in pain.

Dr Srinagesh Simha of Karunashraya, Bengaluru, is no stranger to ill health. 'I was three years old when I decided I was going to be a surgeon. A doctor who was a family friend gave me his old stethoscope and that encouraged me further. I was a successful surgeon, and my wife was an anaesthesiologist. Together we set up the surgery and anaesthesiology departments at Manipal. Then between January 2002 and January 2006, I began to suffer from kidney failure. I had three kidney transplants, and then word was brought to me that my senior was not very sure I should return to surgery because the chance of infection was high. And I remember feeling a sense of relief. But I needed something meaningful to do and there I was, a founder of Karunashraya, so I decided to go into palliative care.'

With his special empathy for those in distress and his interest in spirituality, Dr Srinagesh Simha has struggled with the answer to 'Why me?' and has come to the simple conclusion that 'there is no answer to that. It's a spiritual, existential question and there is no one-size-fits-all answer because each time it is asked, it is a new question. But what I have discovered is that most of the time the person only wants a safe space to vent. At first, I would say, "I can understand" because I had been through the grind of three kidney transplants, but then it was brought to my attention that I was shifting the discourse away from the other person to myself. Then I shifted to "I can imagine", but actually, I discovered that I don't think I can imagine what it must be like to be poor, marginalized, ill, facing death and worried about what will happen to the family after death. So, I now say, "I cannot even imagine", but that is only when I feel I have to say something. Otherwise, I find that quietly listening can help reduce distress. But where the existential distress is severe, we ask a spiritual counsellor from the patient's faith tradition to come in.'

Dr Priya Thomas of NIMHANS, Bengaluru, explains, 'Often professionals like to use statistics or risk factors when a patient asks "Why me?" They add sometimes that we could also ask, "Why not me?" I don't think this approach is very helpful. We should ask the patient if they have any answers that come to their mind when they ask themselves this question. It may be that if they have some guilt or misconceptions about the disease those could then be addressed. It is important for professionals not to shy away or close the conversation when this is asked. It is really an invitation to talk about their fears and their hopes for the future. It is fundamentally a spiritual question and an opportunity to address questions related to the purpose of their life and their feelings about death.'

When Silence Is Not Golden

I am sitting in an office at NIMHANS, Bengaluru, with a doctor and a young man from Tumkur. He has come with his seventy-seven-year-old father who has been diagnosed with acute myeloid leukaemia. The doctor asks whether the family would like to tell him or whether she should tell the patient herself.

The answer is no.

'Would they like to tell him then?'

Another flat no.

'Why not?'

'*Tension mein aayega* (He will get tense),' says the young man.

'Do you think he is not tense now?'

A shrug.

The doctor tries again: 'Imagine you have an exam tomorrow, but you don't know what subject it is. How can you prepare for it?'

'Just walk away, forget it,' the young man says with a victorious smile. The doctor acknowledges defeat.

The question often is: To whom should the doctor break the bad news?

The answer should be simple. This is about the patient's body and the patient has the right to know. Since this is news that will affect the family, the family has the right to know too. This is called collusion.

In medical terms, collusion refers to a situation where healthcare providers, patients or their families withhold information about a diagnosis, prognosis or treatment options, typically to protect the patient from distress.

In many countries, particularly those that emphasize patient autonomy and informed consent, collusion is seen as problematic because it denies patients the right to know about their condition and make informed decisions about their care.

But in India, we are a predominantly collectivist society where family plays a central role in decision-making, especially in healthcare. The well-being of the individual is often viewed as intertwined with that of the family.

And so, in practice, two things often happen here. Either the patient is told the news and asks that the family be kept in the dark or the family is told the news and asks that the patient be kept in the dark.

In the Indian context, doctors are often seen as authority figures, and sometimes as decision-makers rather than facilitators of shared decision-making. Families may pressure doctors to withhold information, and many doctors comply, believing that they are acting in the patient's best interest. This is compounded by the fact that many patients defer to their families and doctors rather than seeking detailed information about their condition.

On condition of anonymity, an oncologist tells me: 'Collusion is common. Everyone does it. But it is the doctor who makes the call about whom to tell.'

'Whom do you tell?' I ask him.

'In the case of minors, it's easy. You tell the parents or the guardian, and you let them take the call. With old people, you tell their children if they have children, or the grandchildren if they have brought the grandparents along. If the person is the earning member, they have to know because they need to plan.'

'Let's just suppose you're the old person and you were brought to the hospital by a grandchild. Would you like to know?'

'Of course,' he answers without hesitation. Then he says, 'I know where you're going with this. But you see, sometimes a patient will actually say: "I don't want to know. Tell my family." Or the patient will say, "Please don't tell my family about this. I will." And there are times when I know they won't, but what can you do?'

'Whoever is given the bad news assumes that the others in the family will not be able to take it,' says Dr Vidya Viswanath of Homi Bhabha Cancer Hospital & Research Centre, Visakhapatnam. 'They think they will have heart attacks and fall over and die. This is what we learn from cinema, at any rate.'

Modern medical ethics see collusion as bad for the patient, the family and all the medical practitioners involved. Dr Kathryn Mannix writes in her book *With the End in Mind: How to Live and Die Well* (2017): 'It can be daunting for a family to discuss bad news. Sometimes if the bad news is broken only to the patient, or only to a family member, that individual can find themselves with the burden of knowing a truth they dare not speak. This can lead to a whole conspiracy of silence that isolates people from each other's strength and support. It is possible to be lonely despite being surrounded by a loving family, as each person guards their secret knowledge for the love and protection of another.'

In a way, collusion means that you can avoid the difficult conversation in its entirety. But information like that can leak.

'Patients know a lot more than families give them credit for,' says Dr Jayarajan Ponissery of Cipla Palliative Care Centre, Pune. They have been taken to TMC, which is known to be a cancer hospital, or they are meeting oncologists – it doesn't take them long to find out what is going on. Or they overhear a telephone conversation.'

Dr Suchi Gaonkar agrees, 'Sometimes a patient will say: "What's wrong with me, doctor?" I generally ask:

"What do you know about your disease?" And they generally say: "I think I have cancer." I ask: "Why do you think that?" And the patient says, "I heard my child talking to the doctor", or "I heard my daughter telling her friend on the phone", or "They looked very sad when they came back with the reports". But if they don't know, I say: "Do you want to know?" Most people say "Yes" but some say, "No. Whatever it is, God will take care of me." And they close down. Sometimes it seems as if hearing the diagnosis is enough to make it real. But those are a minority.'

Dr Anupama Borkar, professor at and head of the medical oncology department, Goa Medical College and Hospital, has a pragmatic approach: 'Collusion is far more common in India than in the West. Here we want to protect our loved ones from bad news. Collusion is not always detrimental. We often see cases of an elderly gentleman or a lady who has stopped making their own decisions maybe a decade ago. The children have taken over decision-making. This person is discovered to have a malignancy, stage 4. You explain it to the children, and they agree to go on palliative care but they ask you not to tell the parent. In that case, there does not seem to be much point in inflicting this information on the patient. It might, in fact, add to their discomfort.'

But there are times when collusion creates a feeling of betrayal. Dr Srinagesh Simha of Karunashraya tells of a man who grew very angry with his family for keeping him in the dark. 'He told them to go away and not come back until he called for them. Over the next three days, he called his lawyer, got his will done, called his accountant and arranged all his financial matters, and once he had settled his affairs, he agreed to see his family again. The upside of letting the patient know is that weddings can be brought forward or garlands exchanged or at least an engagement can happen. But sometimes the patient is brought in so late that none of this is possible. By the time the doctors refer them to us, there's nothing much we can do other than keeping them comfortable,' he says. 'If the patient does not know what is happening and that his care is in palliative mode now, the expectations from the treatment may be unreasonable. This feeling that their health is finally improving is compounded because they begin to feel better because their pain is managed. But then someone, another patient or a caregiver at the institution, may ask innocently, "What cancer do you have?" This can come as a rude shock but now there's nothing to cushion it, no time to plan for the days they have left. They miss out on dealing with the unfinished business of life. They can't, say, make up with an estranged daughter. They can't go and meet the people they want to or see their village one last time. Collusion hurts the patient most.'

When the patient knows, things can be very different. Sameer Cuncolkar from Goa Medical College and Hospital tells me a story about the possibilities of planning when the patient knows the worst and there has been no collusion: 'Some stories stay with you. We had a twenty-nine-year-old patient who had a relapse of cancer. He could have gone in for a bone marrow transplant (BMT), but he could not afford it. His parents were incapacitated for various reasons and could not accompany him to the hospital. One of his brothers was abroad, the other was working somewhere and busy. He would come alone for the treatment and as the disease progressed, he entered the end-of-life phase.

'There was no collusion here; he knew what was happening and got himself admitted at Shanti Avedna, a hospice in Goa. He told us he would like to have a farewell party. It was his last wish. And so, we decided to throw him a real bash. His parents came, and so did one of his brothers. His friends were there and his colleagues. His favourite doctor took time off to show up. His brother was engaged and brought his intended wife with him. He knew he had very little time left, and he wanted to see his brother engaged. The couple agreed, but there were no rings. So we removed the rings from our keychains, and they exchanged these rings in his presence. There were balloons and cakes and singing. That night he passed away.'

Acceptance and Openness

In India, there's no specific rule about how much doctors should tell patients about their condition, so it often depends on the doctor, the situation and what the family wants. But things are starting to change. Groups like the IAPC are encouraging open communication, saying patients have the right to know so they can make their own choices. Medical professionals are finding ways to meet families halfway, talking with them first, helping them see why honesty can be important, and then slowly working towards sharing the truth with the patient in a sensitive way.

Of course, this isn't easy, especially in busy public hospitals where doctors barely have a few minutes per patient. Having those deep, empathetic conversations takes time, and time is something many doctors don't have. But even in those challenging situations, there's a growing effort to make these conversations more open and compassionate, step by step. It's not perfect, but it's progress.

Dr Radha Ghildiyal, professor at and head of the Department of Paediatrics at Lokmanya Tilak Municipal General Hospital, Mumbai, says: 'Delivering difficult news, especially in paediatrics, is an emotional and delicate process. Over my thirty-eight years, I've learned that following certain steps can make it more manageable for families and doctors alike. It starts with preparing – creating a private, supportive space and gently setting the stage for the conversation. Next is understanding the family's perspective and their ability to process the situation. Then comes listening – allowing space for reactions like grief, anger or anxiety without judgement. Responding with empathy and validation is crucial to addressing their emotions thoughtfully. Finally, explaining the realities of treatment or care with honesty, focusing on what can bring comfort and ease suffering, ensures clarity and support. This phased approach helps build trust and makes an incredibly difficult journey more bearable for all involved. I am extremely lucky to have found palliative care and be able to set it up in my tenure here in Sion. Our paediatric palliative care team adopts a holistic approach to disease management and treatment through social activities, pain relief, art therapy, play therapy and informal education.'

Meanwhile, in the halls of Hinduja Hospital, I hear pockets of resistance. A doctor says, 'You know the kind of patient we get. They say, "*Doctor aap hi bataao hum kya karein?* (Doctor, please tell us what to do.)"'

Dr Roop Gursahani replies, 'If you have explained everything and then a family member comes back the next day and says, "*Lekin yeh kab theek ho jaayegaa?* (But when will he get better?)," then you should know your communication has failed. It's on you. The more you do it, the better you get at it.'

Perhaps that may explain the need for someone who will guide the patient through the process. Perhaps that may explain the need for the patient navigator.

7
Patient Navigators

When I meet Rohit at the eight-bedded hospice centre run by CanKids, in Delhi, a bandage covers his left eye, but he is sitting up in bed and reading. Rohit is fourteen and right now he wants to get well so that he can sit for his tenth standard examination next year. So what if cancer has claimed one of his eyes? I think of a poem we learned in school, 'Invictus' by William Ernest Henley:

> *In the fell clutch of circumstance*
> *I have not winced nor cried aloud*
> *Under the bludgeonings of chance*
> *My head is bloody but unbowed.*

I did not think to meet an 'Invictus' in a hospital bed in Delhi but here he is.

Rohit and his father undertook the long journey to AIIMS, Delhi, from a village that is four hours from Patna by bus. At Patna, they got into an unreserved compartment of the train. It was crowded, but since Rohit's eye had been pressed nearly out of his head by the growth, a place was made for him to lie down for some of the long journey. When they arrived at the railway station in Delhi, they were conned out of four hundred rupees by the auto driver.

'When I was paying, a man came and asked me how much I had paid for the auto from the station,' Rohit's father says. 'I told him, and he said we had been cheated. He said when we wanted to go back to the station, we should contact him and he would get us a cheap auto. Then he asked if we had a coupon to go into the hospital. I said we didn't, and he said that we had to buy one from him for a hundred rupees. I was going to give him the money when Rohit went to a security guard and asked whether there was a coupon for admission, and the guard said there was no coupon. I lost heart then. I told Rohit, "These big hospitals are not for us. Let us go home." But Rohit would not listen. He said he would get his operation. He would not go back.'

Rohit powered his way through the maze of AIIMS, his father tells me with obvious pride. It was the boy who found the palliative care team by the simple expedient of asking if there was anyone who would help; it was he who took his father to the social worker who sent them to CanKids; and so in a way, it was he who got the operation done.

I shake the boy's hand and say the words I have found effective: 'I am proud of you, Rohit,' I say in English, and I am rewarded with a huge smile.

'I want to go home,' says Rohit. 'I have to study. We did not bring my textbooks. The didi here gave me some but they are different from the ones in Bihar.'

Every day, thousands of Rohits and their caregivers come from remote villages, travelling to what are called tertiary care centres – big hospitals located in a major city, where specialized expertise and equipment are available.

For those who have covered hundreds of kilometres carrying their burden of disease and of hope, the very architecture of the big tertiary hospital in a city can be intimidating. Sometimes, the campuses are huge, and often there is no indication of where one should begin.

At present India's tertiary healthcare system seems divided into two distinct parts: There are the well-resourced corporate hospitals and there are the overburdened public hospitals. The former are professional and competent, and even attract medical tourists from the West. The latter are understaffed and overworked, and stress levels are high for doctors, nurses, caregivers and even patients. But, against overwhelming odds, public hospitals achieve minor miracles every day: Patients are restored to health at a fraction of the cost of their air-conditioned counterparts.

However, public hospitals are legacy institutions. They have been built in bits and pieces, with departments added on to keep pace with technology, and wards added when funds came through or donors came forward. The result is that even the best-run public hospital can seem like a maze to the first-time patient.

Navigating this maze can be exhausting and defeats both the patient and carer. It can be a cruel experience – nobody's fault but cruel still – at a time when kindness and ease are the greatest need.

YANA – You Are Not Alone

The writer Susan Sontag once pointed out that a disease can isolate the ill person. There is a dreadful feeling of being alone, of being isolated from the kingdom of the well.

'As a person with lived experience, having battled cancer and the depression that came with it, I understand how crucial mental health is in the cancer journey. At CanKids, we are committed to prioritizing mental health as an essential component of cancer care, integrating psychological support into every stage – diagnosis, treatment, survivorship and palliative care,' says Poonam Bagai, the founder of the organization. 'Our goal is to foster patient-centred care that treats the person, not just the disease, while creating an enabling environment for patients and caregivers to voice their concerns and experiences meaningfully.'

She believes: 'When a family hears the words "your child has cancer", their world is forever altered. It's not just about the disease, it's also about the emotional toll, the uncertainty, the sense of loss. At CanKids, this understanding has shaped their work, leading to the creation of the YANA Protocol – *You Are Not Alone.*'

Some of the patient navigators at CanKids are parents who have been on this journey themselves. They know what it's like, they have faced similar situations. Now they have returned to do what they can to help those who are just starting out on this long, hard road.

Patient navigators start as volunteers and become full-fledged team members after extensive training and internships. Their role is simple but vital: to listen without judgement; share their own experiences when it's helpful; and act as a bridge between the family and the hospital staff, explaining medical jargon in a way that they can understand it and finding out what the words mean when they don't, answering questions or getting answers to questions and even helping the families find their way around the hospital.

This isn't just about emotional support, though that's a cornerstone. CanKids recognizes that the challenges families face go beyond their child's medical treatment. The YANA Protocol is holistic, addressing financial support, education, nutrition, hygiene and even logistical needs like navigating hospital departments or finding accommodations.

Where deeper needs arise – when families face depression, overwhelming grief or a sense of hopelessness – YANA ensures access to professional psychological support. The statistics are stark: One in three patients or caregivers struggles with depression during their cancer journey. CanKids responds with a team of psycho-oncologists, trained not just in therapy but also in understanding the unique needs of children and families facing cancer.

The patient navigator works as part of a broader support team. Social workers step in to provide financial counselling and access to government schemes. Psychologists use storytelling, art and play to help children process their emotions. Dieticians ensure families understand how to support their child's treatment with proper nutrition and hygiene. Teachers help children continue their education, recognizing that learning is both a right and a way to hold on to hope.

Each patient navigator or social worker takes responsibility for a specific set of families under the YANA Mera Haath Thaam (hold my hand) programme. They become the family's go-to person for everything – from practical help to emotional support – throughout their journey.

At CanKids, even the smallest details matter. For families travelling far from home for treatment, their 'home away from home' facilities offer not just a place to stay but also a sense of community, a reminder that they are cared for, even in their darkest moments.

The YANA Protocol is more than a programme; it's a promise that no family will face cancer alone. It's a living embodiment of Poonam Bagai's vision – to treat the person, not just the disease, and to create a world where every voice, every tear and every story matters.

In every hospital room, waiting area and counselling session, CanKids delivers one simple but powerful message: *You are not alone. And you never will be.*

The Kevat (Navigator) Programme

As director of TMC, Dr Rajendra Badwe could see how the legendary cancer hospital that had saved so many lives was also a challenge to the patients, their caregivers and attendants because of its architecture and its size.

TMCs are tertiary centres, which means that they are often the last resort for thousands of rural patients who come from all parts of India.

Dr Badwe noticed how difficult the first encounter was for most of these visitors. 'One of the biggest problems is that we do not recognize how alien and terrifying a hospital can be to someone who is visiting it for the first time. We are completely insensitive to this problem. We do not put ourselves in their shoes. I have observed that new patients often display a startle reflex like a baby's. Any loud sound brings on a moment of fear. I have seen how this environment and its complexity can even overshadow the terror of the possibility of cancer, and then we bombard them with treatments, some of which are unnecessary. We throw new information at them every day and expect them to assimilate all this, keep their cool, think rationally and make sensible decisions.'

This extraordinary empathy and compassion led Dr Badwe to conduct a survey with his patients in 2017, asking them about their needs. 'About 3,500 patients were surveyed to understand how they felt about the service we were providing. It is one thing to believe that your service is the best on offer, but surely this must be tested against how the patients perceive it. This survey revealed areas that we have never thought of.'

The responses pointed out the need to bring in palliative care earlier for all-around support. 'Our patients have multiple problems,' says Dr Badwe. 'Sometimes it is about accommodation, sometimes the finance to pay for the treatment. Sometimes money for day-to-day expenses. These patients must face all these problems even while they are handling new decisions every day. If we can smooth some of this away by solving these problems, we have a better chance of starting treatment quickly because their minds can be focused on the treatment plan.'

Then he heard of the Patient Navigator Programme, pioneered in Harlem, New York, by Dr Harold Freeman who found that when people from the community were trained to navigate patients through the hospital, it improved outcomes by 40 per cent. Dr Badwe saw immediately how something similar might help his own patients. And so, the Kevat (or 'boatman') Programme was born. The name is metaphorical, symbolizing the role of a guide who helps patients and their families navigate the often-turbulent waters of advanced illness.

The Tata Memorial website says the Kevat Programme was designed 'to create a taskforce trained to handhold cancer patients and help them navigate through the cancer continuum of diagnosis, treatment, cure, survival; and serve special needs of palliation, end-of-life; to offer seamless care to patients and survivors'.

If you read that carefully, you will mark the word continuum. With many diseases – cancers, non-communicable diseases – the patient and the doctor may make a journey together that lasts for years. If a Kevat is there from the beginning, this journey is made much easier.

The satellite centres are also picking up this idea of navigators. At Dr. Bhubaneswar Borooah Cancer Institute in Guwahati, they are known as 'Suhrids'.

Dr Badwe acknowledges that the project owes much of its success to the involvement of Nishu Goel, head of patient navigation at TMC.

Nishu Goel lost her mother to a virulent oral cancer first identified by a dentist in Kanpur. It was when the cancer recurred that she brought her mother to Tata Memorial and grew interested in how patients navigated the complex system of India's premier cancer hospital.

The Kevat Programme began as a volunteer-driven initiative. 'Much good work was done by volunteers,' Goel says, 'but we felt that there was a need for a more structured environment and a systematic programme of training. It was necessary to train a cadre of people who would go through a formal curriculum instead of relying on what they had learned during their time as patients or caregivers. With the help of Tata Trusts, we devised a course structure of thirty-six credits, open to postgraduates of all fields. A wide variety of people from dental surgeons and nurses to technologists have graduated and become Kevats.'

A Kevat-patient relationship begins at admission but does not end at discharge. 'So many patients who come for follow-up have no idea of the support groups from which they can draw emotional support and learnings,' says Goel.

She points out that Kevats may see 'up to twenty patients on a daily basis, and in order to ensure that the patient gets closure, the Kevat has a target, a defined time within which to find a solution to the patient's problems. A week is the maximum allowed for closure.'

She says, 'All the verticals of a hospital have their own timelines, information and standards, but often they aren't talking to each other. The Kevat becomes your shadow buddy who walks you through the system. There are all kinds of people who come here. There are the underprivileged for whom the hospital is a blessing, then there are those who are entitled and believe that if they are private patients they do not belong in any line. The Kevats must learn to deal with all these.'

With pardonable pride, Dr Badwe talks about the centre in Sangrur, in the heart of rural Punjab: 'Here, we ensure that financial aid is given within half an hour. And this is in the middle of nowhere. A Kevat has to be someone who has the patient's back. We need them to take ownership.'

Dr Badwe adds: 'It takes a clinician to treat but a community to care. There was a huge gorge between the patient and the doctor. The navigator is a bridge across these troubled waters. By being present from the very start, the navigator is looked upon by the patient as part of the multidisciplinary medical team that is trying to help them, but from the doctor's point of view, the navigator is a part of the patient's family. Thus, the navigator should know something about cancer, should have common sense and compassion together with a huge amount of patience.'

No Patient Left Behind

To see the programme in action, I am invited back at TMH, Mumbai, one morning. It is a tumultuous day, as every day is. I end up at the wrong gate, my contact is waiting in another building as if to prove that even if I have visited before, I will still need help navigating this impressive complex. Dr Tanzeem Sayed, who has studied Unani medicine, and Dr Neha Desai, a dentist by training, are the patient navigators who take me through the programme.

Although, technically speaking, the Kevat course is open to anyone with a degree from a recognized university, preference is given to those with some patient or medical experience. What helps also is proficiency in a third Indian language besides English and Hindi because language can often be a barrier in patient communication.

'The common background is empathy,' says Dr Badwe. 'Difficult to find, difficult to judge.'

And this is because it isn't just about the disease; culture plays a major role in care. 'A patient in Varanasi, for instance, would get a date for an operation, and would come back and refuse because he might have been told by an astrologer that the day was not auspicious,' says Dr Neha Desai. 'In another case, a woman was told on the day before her operation that there was a 50 per cent mortality rate. She refused to be operated on. She said that she would not be able to live without her husband and her husband would not be able to live without her. The next day when we went to the ward, she was beautifully dressed and ready to go home. She said she would live out her remaining life with her husband, however long they had. Patient autonomy requires us to respect a decision like that even when we may not agree with it.'

Dr Desai tells me an instructive story: 'I was in Varanasi when there was a hullabaloo in the OPD. When I went to see what the matter was, it was a father and daughter who had come to seek help. The father was feeling suffocated in the air-conditioned precincts of the OPD because there seemed to be no source of air. He had never been in an air-conditioned space before. To add to the chaos, they spoke Bhojpuri and needed interpretation. His daughter taught dance to children in the village and ran a small shop. She had started complaining of pain in her leg, and on examination by some local doctor, had been told that amputation was the only possible solution because there was a growth on the bone. When she was told that a biopsy would be needed, she baulked, refused and threatened to leave. Her father told us he had no way to pay for any treatment, and it was only when we organized five thousand rupees to be given to them that they agreed to the biopsy. On the day of the biopsy, the young woman suddenly took fright at the needle and lost her temper with the doctor. He was surprised because she had been given a local anaesthetic. He lost his cool and told her she could leave if she wanted. Once again, we had to talk the father and daughter into coming back for the biopsy. There was a gap of a few days between the biopsy and the results, and then to our bad luck, the report read: Insufficient tissue sample. It had to be done again, and this had to be explained to the two. And so, another biopsy was done, but the good news was that it was not cancer; it was a tumour but could be treated with injections. This took some doing to explain that the first needles were tests and now this was the cure.'

Dr Sayed adds: 'Tata Memorial serves all kinds of

people from every walk of life. There was once a woman who had a huge mass on her breast. She had a shawl as the only covering for her upper body. I asked her what happened, and she said that the blouse she had no longer fit her. So, we organized some nighties for her and then got them cut and hemmed right there so that she could wear them and sit in peace. In each area, the centre has different problems. In Sangrur, we are in the heart of an agricultural community, and sometimes if there is work to be done or harvesting or sowing, a patient may not turn up for their appointment.'

She continues, 'I remember one case where I was sitting in the OPD when a middle-aged woman came up to me and asked me; "Do you know a place where I can go to die?" I immediately put everything else on hold and sat down to talk to her. It turned out that she had looked after her father who had died of cancer. After his death, she had reclaimed her life. Then she was diagnosed with cancer herself. Her brother refused to help, so she had only her sister and her sister's husband, and she did not want to burden them. I looked at her papers and it seemed she had a fair chance, but even if she had been told this before, she did not see it. She only saw the bag and the stoma and the idea of another traumatic encounter with the healthcare system, with raising funds and bearing side effects, and she wanted nothing to do with it. And so, we found her a place at the Borges Home, and she went peacefully, with her self-respect intact.'

Paving New Pathways

The Kevat Programme has touched many lives. It has shown proof of concept in pure numbers too. The patients follow their doctors' instructions and visit the hospital regularly, becoming allies in their treatment. They report an improved quality of life. Doctors can work more efficiently because the Kevat has taken a medical history, and the doctors know that they can refer associated problems to the Kevat who will steer the patient to the correct department or find help outside.

Dr Vineet Samant, medical superintendent, TMH, says: 'Doctors have always been overworked and that continues to be the case even though we have added nine centres in the past nine years. Unfortunately, although those centres have considerable footfalls, the footfalls here are growing all the time. Therefore, we have two issues: We need clear communication lines between the patient and the clinician, and we need clear communication lines between the centres for system improvement. Kevats bridge these gaps. When they meet the patient, they are the clinician's representative; when they meet the clinician, they are the patient's representative. They join the dots. They have no other responsibilities but to keep this communication going. The medical social workers, for instance, have a great deal of paperwork to get through. The Kevats report to the administration, to the clinicians and to the competent authority.'

Dr Badwe would like to see Kevats spread out in the community at large to help with screening so that cancer can be detected early when there are almost always better prognoses. He says: 'In a study in the Philippines, after screening, it was found that 75 per cent of those diagnosed did not take treatment. Now that defeats the purpose of screening in the first place. Because when we have someone walk into a tertiary centre like a TMC, they already know or suspect that they have a problem. At the screening stage, you are telling people who were going about their normal lives that something might be wrong and they should get it attended to. It's much more difficult to get them to come and start treatment. The Kevat could help bring these patients in early which would mean better outcomes.'

This is only the beginning. There are, at the time of writing this book, a total of eighty active Kevats and Kevat Assistants across the far-flung hub-and-spoke model of the Tata Memorial's ambit. There are 80,000 new patients every year at TMH, Mumbai, alone. 'There are nationally around 1,40,000 new cancer cases that come to us every year. We do about a million follow-ups. That means, of the annual load of 9.3 lakh, we look after 1.4 lakh patients.'

In 2023, the Kevat Programme marked its first international collaboration with a hospital in Indonesia where twenty-one healthcare professionals went through a hybrid course; they had virtual lectures and then came to Mumbai for hands-on experience of the system.

At the time of writing, there are forty seats for which nearly 400 people apply each year.

Dr Sudeep Gupta took over the reins of TMC as its director in December 2023. Over a Zoom call, he tells me that he first heard of palliative care during his medical training at AIIMS. 'We have eleven hospitals now – two are being built – and together we deal with 1,20,000 new cancer cases every year, which is about 10 per cent of the new cases in India. Palliative care is an extremely important component of the three pillars that make up our core commitment – that of service, education and research. We are fully committed to integrating palliative care into the treatment our patients receive at every step of the way.'

Dr Navin Khattry, deputy director of the Advance Centre for Treatment, Research & Education in Cancer (ACTREC), TMC, Navi Mumbai, says, 'It was our good fortune that the Kevat Programme was already mature and nuanced and had proof of concept. When we implemented it at TMC, Navi Mumbai, we immediately saw the benefits in the way the patients responded and the easing of the strain on the team.'

Grief and Guidance: A Mother's Story

At the Maulana Azad Medical College Hospital, Delhi, I chat with Shahnaz Hussein, who has been a patient navigator since 2014. She lost her child to cancer and so she says, '*Main usey in bacchon ke beech dhoondhti rehti hoon.* (I look for him in these children.)'

She began at AIIMS, where she lost her son. 'I often had to visit the ward where I took my son. I could not bear that, so I asked for a transfer.' The children, she says, have a special rapport with her. 'They tell me about their day, they complain about their parents. I think they see their parents telling me things and they feel I must be able to help so they think I might be able to sort out some of their grievances too.'

She does not often tell the parents about her loss. 'I can't do that because it might cause them to lose hope. So, I am careful how I reveal this and when. Often the parents are afraid of the hospital, its vastness, alienness and busyness. They want to take the child and run away. So, we try to calm them down, to reassure them, that all this is here to help you, all this is here for you and your child.'

She takes calls from the parents of her patients even late in the night or in the wee hours of the morning. 'Because if someone has called you at that time, it must be because they are very scared, they are feeling alone or desperate. I cannot ignore them, even the missed calls. I return them,' she says.

Ms Hussein has the marks of a deep sadness somewhere behind the ready smile and the competent manner. And a self-criticality I find rare. When I ask her what is difficult about her work, she says, 'I do not think I can give them the emotional support they need. I can help them with the system, I can explain how to maintain standards of hygiene, I can tell them the importance of nutrition, but I feel somewhere we all need to do much more for them.'

―――

Dr Elisabeth Kübler-Ross and Dr Cicely Saunders both noticed how patients who were no longer curable would be packed away into the far ends of the ward where they were supposed to face death on their own with minimum medical attention.

In India, there are stroke victims who are taken home and left in bed for decades because doctors have said some version of 'There's nothing more we can do for the patient'. Many children who suffer from congenital disorders, especially in rural settings, fall through the cracks of the healthcare system unless they are lucky enough to encounter a health professional who suggests palliative care. With physiotherapy and occupational therapy, for instance, such children may have functional lives. Palliative care might also help the family understand and deal with the situation.

Instead, they and many other patients of degenerative diseases and incurable conditions are told: 'There's nothing more we can do for you.'

'Those are words that should be banned,' says Dr Mary Ann Muckaden, who was a radiation oncologist at Tata Memorial for over thirty-five years. She saw her fair share of patients who had come to her towards the end of their life.

Perhaps this was why, after retirement, she has been working tirelessly for the cause of palliative care.

'There is always something we can do. We may not be able to cure, we may not be able to make the disease or the condition go away, but there is always something we can do. We can help patients live their best lives within the limits of what they are going through. We can listen to them and their families. We can be there for them. That's the essence of palliative care. That we are not here just to cure but also to care.'

8

The Hidden Cost of Caring

'Take Care of Yourself, Kaki!'

Late afternoon, and I am standing somewhere in the northern suburbs of Mumbai waiting for Dr Pranjal Fulbandhe, nurse Anikta Mhatre and social worker Swati Baid. The Palcare team turns up in an autorickshaw and scoop me up, dividing the team into two. Founded in 2015 by Pheroza Bilimoria in memory of her husband, the Jimmy S Bilimoria Foundation, also known as Palcare, offers home-based palliative care services in Mumbai.

On the ride, Dr Fulbandhe says: 'AETCOM is treated as some kind of fun subject. There are classes but nothing that will prepare you for the work, nothing that will prepare you for this kind of day.'

Is it very tough?

'Not tough,' she says, 'but tough too. It is like yoga almost, yoga for the soul. If you wanted to help people when you started out to become a doctor, then this is where you should head. That's what I tell people.'

And then we arrive at a *chawl*, a typically Mumbai construct, a building in which each family has a separate space, generally one or two large rooms but toilets are shared.

Before we go up, Dr Fulbandhe warns me that though the patient is aware that he has cancer, he has not been told it is incurable and that no further treatments have been recommended. The family knows. Is this common? I ask though I already know the answer. Collusion is an Indian epidemic. 'Very,' says Sister Ankita. 'We see it as the family's decision whether they are going to tell the patient or not.'

We enter a one-room-kitchen in which Rama Pawar; his wife Sharada, who is his primary caregiver; his son and daughter-in-law and their child live. Rama himself is lying on a narrow divan against the wall. He seems calm but veering towards the bluer shades of calm. His voice is slow, as if coming through cotton. Dr Fulbandhe kneels down so that her face is on level with his.

The Hidden Cost of Caring

Rama was a poet, a public speaker in his time. Dr Fulbandhe tells him that I am also a poet and asks if he would like to share his poetry. He waves a hand emptily.

His wife says he cannot write these days as his hand trembles.

Sharada is worried about how little he eats: a couple of chapattis, some varan, and he is done. 'You told me give him omelette, give him besan, but he won't touch it,' she says.

The patient's stomach seems swollen and tight. He is retaining water and complains of breathlessness. 'He does not have the courage to sit up,' Sharada says. 'He says he thinks he might get stuck upright.'

He is still able to make it to the bathroom himself, but in the night, he wakes them up.

'I tell him: "Look at me. See how I have to get up. I put an elbow on the ground and push myself up. You can do it, try." But he won't do it.'

The doctor and nurse examine the patient: temperature, blood pressure, blood sugar. All are normal.

What worries them is Rama's sudden decline. On their last visit, he was sitting up. Now he seems to be confined to his bed. Sharada says that he seems afraid of something, perhaps of everything. Perhaps the bed is a refuge. He has become unusually sensitive to sound. He can't bear the television and no longer looks at his mobile. I wonder if it could be that he is afraid of death, but since no one has spoken of it to him, he is unable to talk about it.

The team sits with Sister Ankita, a warm circle of women. Perhaps the nurse senses that the fear may be impending death and she says to the family that it may be time to tell him, but the decision is theirs. She offers support: 'We can tell him together.'

Sharada says that she will consult with the family and let them know.

'Take care of yourself, Kaki,' says Dr Fulbandhe. 'If you fall ill, how will everyone manage?'

Sharada was supposed to have a minor operation but she has postponed it. The doctor assured her that she would be home in a week. 'But how will he manage during that week?'

The team now fears that if he does not get up and change position, he might end up with bedsores. 'Bedsores can be very painful. Oil massages will help avoid them.'

It seems the session is coming to an end when Dr Fulbandhe says, 'What, Kaki? What are you thinking about?'

'About him and ...'

But she can go no further and begins to cry. Dr Fulbandhe moves aside for Swati, the counsellor, who moves in and closes the circle again.

'We won't lie to you. We won't say he is going to get better. He's not. But we can try and support him as long as he is here, right?' Swati asks.

Sharada nods. She tries to pull herself together.

'We all say how much we admire you for all that you do, Kaki, right?'

Nods all around.

'Who knows whether we'll be able to manage at your age.'

Sharada collects herself and speaks. 'Yes, people always say: "How do you manage with this one and your grandchild?" She won't eat unless I feed her. And all this ...'

She puts away her momentary weakness. 'You were talking about bedsores and all, na? So, I got upset.'

'We're not saying he *will* develop them,' Sister Ankita says comfortingly. 'We're saying he *could* develop them over time if you're not careful.'

I am impressed by the fact that the team sits on the ground, but most of all, by the time spent and the gentleness of the team. It is this more than anything else that I think I have cherished in all the hours spent with palliative care teams across the country. We live in a transactional world and one of its first casualties is gentleness because it takes time and it takes a psychic energy that we find difficult to spare. To be gentle with each other, we have to be completely present, and this means putting down everything and staying in the moment with the other person.

Outside, Dr Fulbandhe says, 'I hope they agree to tell him soon. He does not have much time left.'

I wonder whether the poet knows. Our conversation was held not three feet from his bed. His wife's tears, the urgent whispers, his own reluctance to move, all these seem like signs that he does.

But I can also see that the web of trust between the palliative care team is held in place by respect. They must empower and support the caregivers but they must also respect their wishes. Anything less would be a betrayal.

The Love Assumption

The assumption is love. We assume that parents love their children, that children love their parents and that siblings love each other. We assume that the bedrock of the family is love; and this is so often the case that we find departures from the norm shocking, even horrifying. But illness can strain the bonds of family simply because so much changes when a person is ill, especially when the illness is set to last for a long time.

A caregiver is a paid or unpaid person who helps someone who is ill with the activities of daily living. Ashla Rani, a techie who suffered a train accident that confined her to a wheelchair and is now a trustee of Pallium India, remembers that when she arrived at Pallium for the first time, she was impressed by the fact that they were also interested in how her mother was handling the situation: 'My mother was caring for me, cleaning me, bathing me, feeding me. When we came here, she was asked: "What is your name? How did you come to care for her? How do you feel about this?" When she told them about her chronic backache, they asked: "Will you be able to do this by yourself? Do you need help?" I learned so much from that and I use it in my work here, to keep patients front and centre,' Ashla says.

I am reminded of this on a visit to Golden Butterflies, Chennai. The NGO reaches out to all children with life-limiting or life-threatening illnesses.

'But reaching out to a child means reaching out to the parents, and that means reaching out to the family,' says the founder, Stella Matthew. I see what she means when we set off on a home visit with Sister Saranya and Ramalakshmi who heads the projects team. Dr Sabitha, a volunteer, joins us later.

Saif is fourteen years old and weighs thirteen kilos, a frail form in a blue T-shirt and a diaper. He is asleep when we arrive but his mother, Safina, is welcoming and calm. Golden Butterflies has been in touch with her for a while now; Ramalakshmi and Sister Saranya are now familiar fixtures.

'He was a normal child for the first year and a half,' Safina says. 'He sat up, he was saying a few words. Then he had an operation for hernia and the trouble started.'

Saif was diagnosed as having Hunter's disease, a rare condition that affects one in 1,00,000 to 1,50,000 male births.

'I was pregnant with another child when the doctors told me what my son was suffering from and that it would affect his siblings as well,' Safina says. She is a calm and confident woman with a degree in English literature. 'I would have thought twice about another child, had I known.'

Saif's brother shows signs of Hunter's too, but his is a variant that makes him hyperactive, violent and in need of mood control so that he may attend a special school for the deaf. (Hunter's disease affects hearing too.)

Saif has a severe variation. On the last visit, he had a Ryle's tube inserted to feed him. This visit is to check on the tube. Dr Sabitha turns up and the examination begins.

Saif sleeps through it all.

'It has been a long journey,' sighs Safina as Dr Sabitha and Sister Saranya give her boy a gentle going over. They are both pleased to note how well he is being taken care of. There are no bedsores, his teeth are free of caries, his skin is clear. Safina is clearly on top of this, but she admits to having moments when she needs counselling.

'This is the month of Ramzan,' she says. 'So, I have inner peace. But when it is over, I will need to talk to you.'

Ramalakshmi nods understandingly. And suddenly I see the privations of Ramzan in a new light; they are not an imposition on the faithful, they are a source of strength.

'You are managing very well,' says Dr Sabitha, and Safina sighs. Later, I am told that she does the heavy lifting of looking after her two sons, but her husband is by her side. This is so often not the case that I am relieved. Because two are always better than one.

A human being who is ill just wants to go home to the familiar and the comfortable. Palliative care now works to make sure this is possible in as many cases as possible, hence the emphasis on home care and home visits. But this means that there must be someone who is willing to take over the work. Some families can afford paid help in the form of a nurse or a caretaker, but this is expensive. Many families must learn to take care of the day-to-day operations: cleaning a wound and making sure a tube is not clogged. To this end, training is essential, and the palliative care team must work as if it is making the family and the caregiver an extension of itself.

Technology can help. Dr Veronique Dinand of Wadia Hospital, Mumbai, says: 'One of the good things about COVID-19 was that it made Zoom and other platforms popular. We use Zoom to teach patients self-care, to train parents and caregivers for things like how to manage breathlessness using simple exercises, and to train parents in skills like providing gentle physical therapy or positioning a bedridden child to prevent bedsores.'

Caregiver Burnout

It is not only the patient who wants to weep and sob. It is also the caregiver who often rides a roller coaster of emotions. She – and as we have noted, it is more often than not a woman – is expected at all times to be doing her duty to the best of her abilities, to be on top of everything, to do all this and the other things expected of her because she loves the person. But this love can get corroded over the long haul of an illness.

And that brings us to caregiver burnout, 'a state of physical, emotional and mental exhaustion that happens while you're taking care of someone else. Stressed caregivers may experience fatigue, anxiety and depression.'[5] Also guilt and anger and a host of other feelings. It's a sneaky thing. You might not even notice you have it and then someone says something, and you find yourself in a fit of rage or a storm of tears or both.

When Shaista N. tells me her story, we are sitting in her home in Mumbai. Her father is in the room next door, now almost completely bedridden. He has been suffering from Parkinson's disease for close to two decades and his daughter, once an advertising executive, now works from home, selling insurance. She has borne the brunt of caregiving for several years.

Then she found a support group at the hospital and made friends. It was at one of those meetups that she met another woman, a mental health professional, who had a mother who had Parkinson's. They became friends and began visiting each other.

'One day, she came over and said to me: "It's okay to be angry with your Dad." Immediately, it came to my mouth, "I'm not angry. How can I be angry? He is suffering from this disease the most. How can I be angry?"

'But she just looked at me and said nothing and I began crying and crying. And I remember thinking,

"She has a kind face" and that made me cry all the more. She did not say, "Don't cry", and I remember thinking, why isn't she saying this, why isn't she saying "Don't cry"? Everyone says it. Why isn't she saying it? Now I think she was right not to say it because you have to cry. I cried so much I thought I would vomit. But then it stopped, and I said, "Sorry, sorry." She said, "Strong people also need to cry." And I said, because I was so ashamed I was crying, "Which strong people cry?" She looked puzzled for a moment and said, "Amitabh Bachchan. He cried in every movie." And I started laughing and it was so good. I don't think I had laughed since the time Papa fell and broke his leg when he tried to walk without the ward boy and ended up in the bed.

Then I said, "Shee! I'm shameless, laughing." And she said, "Would Papa not want you to laugh?" And I began crying again, but when I went into his bedroom, Papa asked, "What were you laughing about?" I told him and he also smiled. I realized that I had not given myself permission to feel anything. I saw that I was sad and I was angry and I missed my old life, my colleagues, going to an office and meeting people and not sitting by the phone with half my attention directed at the other room. She gave me the key: You can cry. You can laugh. It's okay. It's life.'

'A serious illness does not just affect the patient, it also impacts the whole family,' says Digambar Sathe, senior homecare social worker at the Cipla Palliative Care Centre, Pune. 'As soon as treatment for the patient starts, it's just as important to support the family and caregivers. They play a huge role in the patient's care, and if they're overwhelmed or burnt out, it can affect how well the patient is looked after. Early support helps families and caregivers handle tough decisions, stay strong, and avoid hitting a breaking point. Taking care of the patient and the caregiver goes hand in hand. If the family is prepared for what's coming, it makes the whole journey smoother for everyone.'

Caregivers find themselves enmeshed in the mechanics of caring. In between bathing and cleaning and assisting with toilet routines, preparing special food and feeding, making sure medications are taken, cleaning feeding tubes or colostomy bags, transporting the patient for tests and visits, and explaining what is going on to friends and family, there is little time to acknowledge the humanity of the patient but even less to acknowledge one's own humanity.

Dr Ambika Rajvanshi, CEO, CanSupport, says, 'If caregivers are emotionally or physically drained, it's hard for them to give quality care, and they can burn out quickly. Simple things like watching a film or having a meal together can give them a much-needed break and help recharge their emotional batteries. It's not selfish – it's necessary. As healthcare providers, we need to remind caregivers that taking out time for themselves doesn't make them any less dedicated to their loved ones. In fact, it helps them be better caregivers in the long run. We have to remind them that looking after their own well-being is just as important as looking after their loved ones.'

Stronger Together: Support Groups

'If you can come together with others who have been there or who are going through the same things, life does not seem so harsh,' says Anuradha Karegar of Wadia Hospital for Children, Mumbai. 'That is why we run a number of support groups.'

On 15 November 2024, something extraordinary happened at the thalassemia daycare centre in the hospital's Haemato-Oncology Ward. Sixteen teenagers, boys and girls, all living with thalassemia major, part of a group they've proudly named 'Star Parivar', gathered together in a vibrant, noisy swirl of energy and emotions. This was a boisterous lot – laughing, joking and sharing pieces of themselves in ways only they could understand.

Thalassemia major isn't just about the biology of a condition; it's about the toll it takes on every aspect of life. It is a severe genetic blood disorder where the body doesn't produce enough haemoglobin, the protein in red blood cells that carries oxygen. Without regular blood transfusions every two to four weeks these kids can't survive. And while the transfusions keep them alive, they come with a heavy price: iron overload, which can damage vital organs. That's where the demanding regimen of iron chelation therapy comes in, removing the excess iron but placing a heavy burden on both the body and the mind.

This isn't a condition that ever takes a break. It's unyielding: the fatigue, the constant hospital visits, and the deeply personal questions that surface – *Why me? Why is my life different?* And while BMT is the only known cure, it remains an option out of reach for most. The process is complex, requires a perfectly matched donor and is often prohibitively expensive. For many families, the emotional and financial strain of even considering a BMT feels insurmountable.

A peer group like this is pure alchemy. It turns isolation into connection, vulnerability into resilience. I meet Dhriti who nailed the Science Olympiad – one of the fifteen in her class and the only one with a life-limiting illness to achieve this. Then there is Shivang, whose YouTube channel shows off his insane sketching skills. Avinash, a football star, plays for his church team with a kind of grit that could inspire anyone to lace up their boots. And Purvi, who tells us about the time she went through a morning transfusion and then absolutely aced her tenth-standard board exam that same day.

Parents are there too, chiming in with their own stories – sometimes joyful, sometimes fraught. Sheila talks about how her teenage son flat-out refuses to take his meds now because, well, teenage rebellion is universal. Bina, meanwhile, has nothing but gratitude for the staff at the hospital. 'They treat our kids like their own,' she says, 'but will the same care continue at the new transfusion centre?' That question hangs in the air, a quiet reminder of the uncertainties they all live with.

For these teenagers, the transition from paediatric care to adult care represents a seismic shift in their lives. At the paediatric day care centre, they've grown up with a network of familiar doctors, nurses and caregivers who know their names, their histories and their quirks. The centre has been a constant source of emotional and medical support – a safe haven where they've felt seen, cared for and understood.

But now, as they step into adulthood, they're moving to adult healthcare facilities that are larger, busier and often less personalized. The intimate bonds they've formed with their paediatric care team will inevitably give way to a new system where they'll need to advocate for themselves more than ever. It's a daunting transition, one that can leave them feeling adrift and overwhelmed. This is where the peer support group becomes not just helpful but also essential. It's a bridge between the old and the new, offering a space where these teens can share their fears, ask questions and find encouragement from others who are navigating the same uncharted waters.

The Power of Shared Journeys

What if you move the emphasis on living with a serious illness from surviving to thriving? How would one do that? Where would one draw strength from? Would it help to meet others who have been there, done that and are still standing tall? 'If they can do it, so can I,' might be a powerful thought. And maybe, just maybe, it's about knowing that when life gets tough, your tribe has your back. Because sometimes, that's all you need to face whatever comes next.

Harmala Gupta of CanSupport was an NRI based in Canada, working on her PhD thesis at McGill University, Montreal, when she was diagnosed with Hodgkin's lymphoma, a cancer of the lymphatic system. It was when Harmala Gupta returned to India that she saw the need for support groups. In 1991, she founded the first peer-based cancer support group in India: Cancer Sahyog in Delhi.

'I am a great believer in support groups, and one of the first things I wanted to do when I returned from

Canada was to start a support group for people with cancer. I approached a few oncologists. The first thing they said to me was, "In India we don't need support groups because we have family. In the West, they have no family." You know, it's funny how we have these ideas about different societies and people. So, I said, "First of all, that's not true. In the West also, they have families and families who are very concerned and want to look after their ill. And secondly, I said, in India, because your caregivers do not have the knowledge, do not have the training, they don't know how to react. It's much worse here. They need support. Yes, the person with cancer needs support but so do the caregivers. So actually, you need two kinds of support groups. You need one for the person who is going through the disease and one for the family.'"

It takes me back to the caregivers' support group meeting I attended at the Cipla Palliative Care Centre, Pune. The caregivers' meeting is held in a community space called 'Dhyaana Dhaarana', a large community space that holds a small library. When I join the meeting, the conversation seems general. Someone says he is surprised that Cipla's centre isn't better known. Tell people about it, he is urged by the team, but you have to be clear about informing them about what we do or else it will raise the wrong hopes. Someone is advising everyone else not to cry or complain. 'What good does it do?' she asks and there are nods, serious nods. Someone says that the patient she is caring for complains about the smallest things: My sister in Kolhapur doesn't call me, why doesn't she call? Again, serious nods, these are things they have all been through. Stories are shared of a 105-year-old woman who is being cared for by her 75-year-old son who had not married for her sake. The mood is approving: *Seva* (selfless service) is valued highly in India.

Community is not about solving problems, it is about hanging the problem out to air and allowing oneself the luxury of admitting that love is a problem, that it makes you vulnerable, that you're hurting, and that you wish you could find an easier way for all this to happen. Only those walking with you or those who have walked this path before can understand the potent mix of emotions that you feel.

Caregiver burnout is a human response, but it need not be inevitable. You need to have some space and time to call your own. You need a group that understands the specifics of your situation. You need peers to tell you that they did it wrong too and it wasn't the end of the world. You need to know you're not alone in the world. That's where a support group comes in. Many support groups meet in person because it allows them to step out of the house but also because it is possible to actually hug someone, offer a tissue, or just pat a hand. But where that's not possible, support groups meet online and find help and sustenance from a screen. In short, palliative care is not just for patients, it's equally for their caregivers too.

You may call me a dreamer but I'm not the only one. Here is my definition of the empowered caregiver.

The doctor breaks the bad news. The patient and the caregiver have time to absorb this and then the patient or the caregiver asks: 'So when do we meet the palliative care team?'

Self-care for Medical Professionals

The overall impression I got from the palliative care

teams was that they found the work deeply satisfying. Responses ranged from 'like a form of meditation' to 'the most satisfying work I have ever done'. And yet palliative care brings one up against death again and again. That cannot be easy.

If the palliative care team is to be effective, it must know the family at some very deep level. It must know about the brother's gambling problem and the father's dependency issues. The patient must feel free to cry and to shout, and the team must allow for these emotions. Roles may be blurred among the team, leading to some confusion and mixed messages. The patient must share deep-seated fears and the highest hopes and all this only creates a strong relationship which is then ended by death. All this can lead to the team itself asking some fundamental questions of its own belief systems.

Dr Priya Thomas of NIMHANS says, 'We do see death as part of the continuum of life, a natural end-point, and not as a failure. But there can be some desensitization to death too. A friend who works in palliative care says she is no longer able to respond to death. That she cannot is worrying her. She is now seeking treatment for it and support is required. You can also develop compassion fatigue, difficult for you as a professional and for the patients too.'

Michelle Normen of Karunashraya says that self-care is an important part of the regular agenda. 'We debrief regularly as a team and draw some healthy boundaries with our cases. This is easier said than done because human beings are involved. Someone may trigger memories. Some other patients may have instant rapport with a medical health professional. Confidentiality can be a huge concern. They may need to share things that might be seen as scandalous, but we must remain non-judgemental.'

Palliative care is one of those fields that defies simple definitions. On the one hand, it's often called the most rewarding branch of medicine. On the other, it's also known for having high burnout rates. Both statements might be true.

Curious about how professionals navigate this intense yet fulfilling journey, I decided to ask some of them: What gets you through? Their answers were thoughtful, honest, and a little unexpected:

- Compassion, they said, but not just for others – it's vital to have some for yourself too
- Acceptance – of your imperfections, your mistakes and the occasional reality that you can't fix everything
- Empathy – not just understanding the problem but also recognizing the person at the heart of it
- A sense of humour because sometimes, laughter is the best way to keep going
- A supportive work environment where you can talk, vent, and share the weight of the job
- Regular timeouts – holidays, hobbies and passions outside of work to recharge
- A family that gets what you do and values it
- A journal for those moments of joy – a successful intervention, a patient's smile, a family's gratitude

And finally, they said, the small victories: the patient who smiles after days of pain, the family who finally feels at peace. Those moments? They're the reason they show up day after day.

Turns out, the secret to surviving and thriving in palliative care isn't a single big thing – it's a hundred small things that keep your heart steady and your hope alive.

Driven by Purpose

All this is different from standard medical practice, which sometimes looks at the body of the patient as a machine that has broken down and needs some repairing. The palliative care team looks at the patient in their setting. They set themselves the task of alleviating all pain, starting with the physical but moving on to the psychological, the social, the economic, the spiritual … This is magnificent. But sometimes I would think: 'You guys are committing to the improbable in a country like India.' Pain seems to be our natural lot. Suffering seems to be a necessary concomitant. How can you set your standards so high? Isn't that like asking to fail?

But then Dr Roop Gursahani explains it to me. When I suggest that there is no way you can think of palliative care in India without a systemic rehaul – a rehaul of mindsets (so that a girl child will be given the same chance at life as a boy child), of public facilities (so that there is clean water and sanitation for all), of inequality (so that no poor parent is ever told, 'Fatten up your malnourished child and bring her back so we can heal her') – Dr Gursahani nods his head in agreement. It is a wide remit, he says. And then he adds: 'You focus on the patient in front of you. That's it. Everything comes down to that.

It reminds me of a story that I find most useful.

A man is walking down the beach. Ahead of him on the beach, he sees hundreds of starfish that have been washed ashore and are stranded. They are dying. He walks a little further, and there is a little boy who is walking amongst the starfish, picking up one and throwing it back into the sea, picking up another and throwing it into the waves, picking up a third, and so on. The man asks, 'What are you doing?' The boy says, 'Throwing them back into the water.' And the guy says, 'There are so many. What does it matter?' The boy bends down and picks up one and says, 'It matters to this one.' So, finally, 'You do what you can,' says the good doctor. 'At some level you have to say that this is all I can do. You have to be kind to yourself. But within those limits, you have to do all that you can.'

And yes, they do commit to the improbable, India's palliative care providers. But what they often do is pull off the impossible: helping the patient accept the limitations of the disease, make up for lost time, restore peace inside, reach out to mend bridges, accept mortality as part of what makes the time we have here so special. Sometimes all of this does not quite happen according to the script. But a lot of it does, in some measure, and often. And every bit of relief, every little comfort and reassurance, every shred of dignity restored is a lifeline.

9

Integrating Palliative Care into Healthcare

If it takes a village to bring up a child, it takes a community to make healthcare a reality. Dr M.R. Rajagopal of Pallium India points out that this is a truth universally acknowledged: 'All over the world, the learning has been that palliative care can only succeed in partnership with general healthcare. And general healthcare for all can only be possible if it is healthcare within the community.'

Where the palliative care system is patient owned and driven, the figures show that the need for palliative care is not limited to cancer patients. The majority of the cases are not cancer related and represent a spectrum from stroke patients to renal failure and children with developmental difficulties. All of them had benefited from palliative care, which has involved the community.

One day every hospital, nursing home and primary healthcare centre will offer palliative care. The community will own it, the patient will look for it, the caregivers will demand it. But that's some way in the future. Right now, the path seems strewn with hurdles. There are, however, examples of palliative care being integrated within community and government hospitals that shine a light on its transformative power in healthcare.

Malathi's Story

As Dr Rajagopal tells Malathi's story, I'm caught in its web. This is the brutal darkness of poverty; darkness made even more stark by the green-flecked gold of a Kerala afternoon.

When morning broke, Malathi roused herself. It was still dark outside, but it was time for her to get up. The octogenarian limped past her grandsons – four young men – and their mother, all asleep. She would now have a bath and set out to the wholesale market, some miles away, buy vegetables and take them to a spot in the local market where she would sell them. Meanwhile, her daughter would wake the four young men up and begin the morning ritual of bathing them, changing them, and helping them clean themselves, even as she kept an eye on the rice gruel that she had set to boil. All four of her sons had a congenital neurological defect that left them with intelligent minds in disobedient bodies. When the gruel was ready and cool, she would drag the young men to a wall, prop them up against it, and feed them, holding their twitching heads still, ignoring an occasional, unintentional flap from a flailing arm.

A routine day for the family.

But that evening, the matriarch Malathi called a family council. It was time to talk, she said. For more than three decades, she had run the house and generally managed to keep things going. She was the pivot on which the family turned, and the pivot was now wearing out.

Malathi looked at the faces turned towards her.

'Tell us, Amma,' said her daughter. 'Tell us what is in your heart.'

Malathi nodded. She knew that the young doctor in the district hospital had taken a look at the twitching and flailing boys, unable to sit up or move, and had labelled them 'mentally retarded'. But she knew her grandsons' brains were not compromised. They understood what was spoken around them, they could make decisions about their future. She loved her grandsons, and now she was placing a choice before them.

For Malathi's body was betraying her. Soon, she would be too old to work, and rather than let the boys live with indignity, she had a suggestion. She would get hold of poison, and they would all kill themselves.

'Malathi asked her family to vote,' Dr Rajagopal continues. 'The boys' mother voted for death. One by one, three of her sons followed suit – they voted for death too.'

But the fourth held out. He voted to live.

'In her mind, Malathi had given each one of them something like veto power,' Dr Rajagopal tells me. 'One of them said he wanted to live, and so they would all live.'

Malathi soldiered on. Her work took a toll on her spine and she suffered a disc prolapse. She needed surgery but she could not take the time off for it. She began to walk with a limp. The nerve damage made her incontinent and this led to frequent urinary infections.

When Malathi died, there were five young men

in that single room. For she had brought home a schizophrenic nephew to live with her, presumably on the assumption that if you were looking after four, one more would not matter.

'Before she died, we had invited her as the chief guest to one of our functions and given her an award for bravery,' Dr Rajagopal says, his gentle voice full of remembered emotion. 'One by one, the rest of the family also died. Only the young man who voted for life remains, and his cousin who is schizophrenic. We are going to visit them today.'

We are driving from Thiruvananthapuram through a lyrical monsoon landscape. It has rained in the morning, so the golden light is strained through wet foliage and the scent of damp earth seeps in through the windows of the car. Here again, it seems that every prospect pleases but only the living conditions of human beings born in poverty can be vile.

When Dr Rajagopal and his team of palliative care workers first visited the family some years ago, they found that the four young men had open wounds on the backs of their heads.

'They were sitting against a rough wall and from time to time, driven by muscular spasms, they would bang their heads against the wall. So, we cleaned and bandaged the wounds and then had a mattress pinned to the wall.'

It is a breathtakingly simple solution to a long-standing problem. But I ask the obvious question: Did they not think of moving them into care?

'That was our first thought. We told them, "We will take you to a home. You will be looked after there." They all said no. They wanted to be in their own home. We respected that.'

Kindness can take many forms, and sometimes it is as simple as a mattress pinned on a wall and a respect for the wishes of the person you think needs help. But it can also take complex forms that require media attention, public interest and governmental intervention. The media covered the young men's story, and the government responded.

'At the time of Malathi's death, there was a very proactive healthcare minister in Kerala. And so, a carer was hired for them,' Dr Rajagopal continued. 'She has been here for years.'

Funds were found to build two more rooms. A television was installed, and that took away some of the tedium. A homecare team from Pallium India would visit regularly to keep an eye on things. The car comes to a halt. Dr Rajagopal looks out. 'Ah, here's Hassan.'

Hassan is a middle-aged man in a shirt and a lungi. He greets Dr Rajagopal with a bright smile and brings him up to date. He has all the papers on his phone and pulls them up, one after the other; he knows every detail of the case. 'Hassan is a neighbour, a friend. He is a volunteer,' says Dr Rajagopal. 'But he is also a hero. In Kerala, the volunteers are the heroes of palliative care.'

Meanwhile, the carer tells Rajiv, the man who has driven us here, that the fan in one of the rooms is not working. Rajiv asks for a stool to see if he can fix the problem. 'We do not have drivers,' says Dr Rajagopal. 'We have palliative care assistants.'

Rajiv climbs on to a stool and unhooks the fan to repair it. On this sultry Kerala afternoon, I can see how this could fit into the mandate for palliative care.

The young man, the man who chose life, is given a gentle but thorough examination. He talks to Dr Rajagopal. They discuss politics and the state of the nation. His television keeps him well informed.

Palliative care is not just a medical intervention but also a compassionate partnership between families, communities and organizations, creating a safety net where every life is valued and every voice matters.

From the Ground Up in Telangana

When I visited Hyderabad, I was told to meet Dr Gayatri Palat, who is a trustee of PRPCS and head of department, Mehdi Nawaz Jung (MNJ) Institute of Oncology and Regional Cancer Centre, Hyderabad. At the hospice run by PRPCS, I meet first with J.N. Jagannath, president of PRPCS, who retired from the Indian Railway Traffic Services. His wife Girija was also in the civil services. When she was chief commissioner of income tax in Nagpur, she was diagnosed with colon cancer stage 3B. She underwent twenty-seven chemotherapy cycles and endless radiation at Apollo in Hyderabad, Lilavati in Mumbai and even Harvard Medical, where a friend was working.

Mr Jagannath shares: 'She had three surgeries, and after the third, I went on long leave to care for her. She was a woman who was full of life. She would say that if there's a one in a million chance, I should like to be that one who makes it ...'

It was when Mr Jagannath was on long leave and was at their home in Jubilee Hills that he heard of PRPCS and met Dr Gayatri Palat. 'Girija died at fifty-eight, and I began to understand what this end-of-life care was like, how excruciating cancer pain can be. I watched my vibrant, intelligent wife as her life ebbed away.'

After he retired as general manager, he did not choose the usual route of the civil servant at sunset: consultancies and seats on boards. 'I came here and said I would like to help those who were facing the same issues.'

He met with Dr Palat and team, and in 2007, PRPCS became an NGO. By a change in government policy, an AIDS centre had to be closed down, and the 52-acre plot left for it by a deceased lady for charitable purposes was made available to PRPCS for a hospice.

Dr Palat joins us and picks up her story: 'I was an anaesthesiologist with a deep interest in pain management. The head of my department was Dr Rajagopal, and so I grew interested in his work. Then an organization based in Vancouver, Canada – Two Worlds Cancer Collaboration – said that they would like to fund palliative care in other states. And so, we wrote letters to many states and promptly we got a reply from Dr B.V. Rao, of the MNJ Institute of Oncology here in Hyderabad. Dr Rajagopal asked if I would move here for a year to pilot the project, and here I am, seven years later.'

Dr Palat has had an amazing run in Telangana. She works with the Government of Telangana and there is now a palliative care programme in each of the thirty-three districts of Telangana. In terms of human resources, each district has one doctor, one physiotherapist and five nurses. 'We also have supportive homecare services, which means we have opioid medications to make sure our patients are kept free of pain.'

In many ways this is a radical shift because it means that patients who come to Hyderabad to be treated in a tertiary centre can go back home, to their districts, to their villages, in between treatment or when it is over. 'We then refer them to a palliative care team in their district, and this means that they will continue to get care and support and access to pain medication, where necessary, in the district centre closest to their homes.'

In addition, the Accredited Social Health Activists (ASHA workers) and the Auxiliary Nurse and

Midwives (ANMs) at the primary healthcare centres have been given some basic training. This will help them recognize the patients who might need palliative care so that they might inform the palliative care team. And while the districts are focusing on cancer, Dr Palat confidently predicts that the demand will change the matrix. 'In general, we have seen that when we look at a population that needs palliative care, about 30 per cent will be patients who have cancer, and 70 per cent will be patients who have other health conditions that make them need assistance. Once they have been factored in – the patients who have had strokes and are bedridden, the ones with cardiovascular or renal conditions, neurological disorders, congenital issues – the scope is huge.'

What makes this especially significant is that it is a sustainable model that does not depend on finding donors. The whole of it has been incorporated into the government health system. 'The challenge now lies in monitoring and evaluation because maintaining quality is always a problem, and in the public healthcare system, it is particularly marked,' Dr Palat says. But it all begins with recognizing what palliative care is, what the needs are and how the care should be delivered.

'A massive sensitization and training programme has been undertaken at every level of the healthcare system,' she says.

Thus, revolutions begin: one state at a time.

Upskilling Community Health Workers in Goa

Dr Ira Almeida explains how the Compassionate Communities programme has taken off over the last year across six panchayats in South Goa. She said: 'It is great to see the community health workers, who we have trained and have regular refresher courses for, working alongside the palliative care teams, as they can then follow up with patients and identify new patients with complex symptom burden. We have trained them to use a scale that identifies community members with serious illnesses who require palliative care. The sarpanch now provides transport logistics for those patients who require to be brought to the primary healthcare centre or the district hospital for further support.

I visit three homes along with the team and witness the power of community work in action – all three patients have suffered strokes and their movement is limited. Sister Renuka, a trained nurse, is a community health worker in the village; she meets us at the local school. We then go together for the visits. The physiotherapist of the palliative care unit demonstrates to the caregivers the exercises that need to be done twice a day. She also teaches Sister Renuka how to monitor the progress and tells each family what signs to look out for to notice the change in movements. Sister Renuka will now follow up every week and knows she can connect with the palliative care team for any support.

I listen as Shraddha, the caregiver to her eighty-year-old mother, thanks the team for bringing a smile to her mother's face that morning. Dr Almeida concludes: 'We have lots more to do, but it is encouraging to see change – one life at a time.'

Integrating Palliative Care into Neurology

Dr Priya Thomas is proud that the first step has been taken to set up a palliative care unit at NIMHANS, Bengaluru.

She says: 'While we always had rehabilitation services, we did not have a unit that followed up with patients, coordinated their care, answered their questions, offered to visit their homes or provided them with mobility support if required. The palliative care unit they have now is doing exactly this.'

Dr Gargi, the project coordinator, explains: 'The department approached Cipla Foundation in 2021 to set up an OPD service to focus on the palliative care needs of patients with dementia (progressive intellectual difficulties), Parkinson's (progressive movement disorders) and ALS (muscle stiffness and difficulty eating). Over 3,500 patients have received care from the unit over three years. 'The feedback from caregivers is motivating for our team to give their best and ensure we deliver the best quality of care.'

At the NIMHANS OPD, I meet Shiva, the caregiver for his seventy-five-year-old wife who has advanced Parkinson's. He has come with his wife as she has concerns about her eating. Dr Kritika, the palliative care physician, focusses on symptom relief and dealing with the patient's discomfort, including medication adjustments, helping Shiva to formulate a home-based plan of care for medical symptoms. Sagarika, the nurse practitioner, discusses with Shiva how he needs to care for himself and that he needs to reach out for assistance when he feels overwhelmed with the situation. She explains how his wife's breathing patterns would likely change over the next few months as well as her sleep pattern, where she may sleep for longer stretches.

Robin, the physiotherapist on the team, explains the importance of movement and demonstrates exercises that need to be done at home sitting up and lying on a bed. They are also introduced to the speech therapist and the occupational therapist who say that they will visit the family over the next fifteen days. The speech therapist will start helping them both with nonverbal communication and easier verbal communication in terms of single words rather than sentences, so that her distress would be reduced in case she loses her ability for verbal communication.

The occupational therapist speaks to the family about how she will visit to assess the family home to reduce the risk of falls by suggesting any simple modifications as well as to make sure Shiva's wife is using her walker properly while balancing her weight.

Dr Priya adds that the social work team will continue to do their psychosocial assessments for the family and continue to offer support to both Shiva and his wife to adapt to the disease as well as manage emotions of anger, fear and guilt while dealing with changes in function and the increased dependency of Shiva's wife on him.

Dr Priya says she hopes that the palliative care unit at an apex government institution like NIMHANS will build a body of evidence for the facilitators and barriers to implementing a palliative care service with patients with neurological conditions. 'We would like to spend the next year disseminating the protocols we have tested over the last two years so that patients with neurological conditions can receive the best possible care, especially in public settings,' Dr Priya says.

In a Kalwa Hospital, a New Start

In Chhatrapati Shivaji Maharaj Hospital in Kalwa, a city adjacent to Thane, Maharashtra, the municipal corporation has taken over the palliative care unit. It has a dynamic team that has taken the project to its heart. The doctors, the nurses and the social workers have all made it their cause.

Dr Pradnya Talawadekar, who leads the palliative care team, tells me that Chhatrapati Shivaji Maharaj

Hospital is a tertiary care centre that serves a large tribal area. 'Most of the children come from underprivileged families,' she says. 'One chronically ill child can upset the whole family's ecosystem. Ours is the first government centre to offer palliative care for non-cancer-affected children.'

Dr Talawadekar attributes part of the success to a nurse, Sister Vijaya Kadam, and the social worker, Rita Moras, who made the project their own. 'Rita and Sister Vijaya Kadam were a magnificent team,' says Dr Swapnali Kadam, now vice dean at the hospital.

It wasn't easy at first. Patients would not listen to them. But that's also understandable. Think for a moment of the caregiver who has brought an ill child into the Kalwa OPD. She – and often it is a woman alone, a mother or grandmother – has just set aside the responsibilities of the household to make this journey. She has probably had to spend some money to get to a railway station and then carry the child up and down endless flights of steps. She now enters the strange, clamorous world of the hospital where all is alien. Everyone is busy and overworked. Everyone speaks in acronyms and when they expand the acronyms, the result is even more challenging.

Hospitals also attract their fair share of scamsters and con artists. Some talk loudly of miraculous cures, hoping to attract the attention of desperate patients or family members. Others make direct approaches. Patients learn defensive tactics.

'So, when we would talk to patients, they would turn away or ignore us,' Ms Moras recalls. 'Just to get their information was difficult.'

Who were these people approaching them with more forms to fill? What could they possibly do? Most patients in Kalwa or in most municipal hospitals are used to waiting for hours in a queue just to see a doctor. Who could these people be who were promising speed and efficiency and talking to them as equals? They couldn't be real.

But Ms Moras and Sr Kadam were not to be deterred by cold shoulders or even hostility. 'If you put yourself in their shoes, then you understand,' says Ms Moras. 'Life has not been easy.'

The turning point came when another nurse, Sister Shivani, gave them a place to sit in the OPD. They were beginning to gain some traction when COVID-19 hit. The palliative care team swung into action, making sure patients stayed in touch, sourcing medicines and, in some cases, even delivering them.

'But one of the doctors said, "Your whole palliative care thing is over now. You can go home and sit there like everyone else,"' Ms Moras remembers. Then she adds with a glint in her eye, 'Today the same doctor sends us lots of patients.'

Ms Moras trained under Dr Mary Ann Muckaden at TMH, Mumbai, chosen out of seventy-five applicants for the vacancy, she says with pride. She worked there for years and then took a break to have a baby. Now she's back and is a force to reckon with.

'Children come in and ask, "*Rita Aunty kahaan hai?* (Where is Rita Aunty?)",' Dr Talawadekar says with a smile. 'I feel a dedicated team of palliative care workers guided by a good mentor can really make a difference.'

Ms Moras looked beyond the patients to the caregivers and beyond the caregivers to the families they came from. There were women who couldn't come to the hospital with a sick child until their mother-in-law said they could go. There were others who walked for hours and hours, carrying a child to save bus fare. And so, when they formed support groups in Kalwa, they didn't just share experiences and support each other, they also formed self-help groups with small amounts of money to give the women some form of economic independence.

At Kalwa, we are talking extended timelines, for, as Dr Talawadekar points out, 'We could be seeing a patient for ten–fifteen years.'

But these are bonds that deepen and mature. And they have given rise to a mature project. Dr Shailija Potdar, the head of the paediatric department, is extremely proud of the project. She adds: 'After six years of this project, the Thane Municipal Corporation has seen the value we add to the quality of life of children and their parents. We now have a full-time dedicated doctor and nurse for palliative care supported by the corporation.'

If it can happen in Kalwa, it can happen anywhere in the country.

It is the beacon on the hill.

Keeping the Momentum Going

The spark to integrate palliative care within the healthcare system has been ignited. Anurag Mishra, head of Cipla Foundation, explains that in the last year, several states that did not have palliative care policies, such as Rajasthan, Karnataka, Himachal Pradesh, Goa and Odisha, have reached out to the Foundation to help with training and delivery of palliative care services through the National Programme of Palliative Care. He says, 'Bringing palliative care to underserved areas like Lucknow, Bikaner and Muzaffarpur, and expanding to public health hospitals and non-oncological conditions is a transformative leap forward. At the Cipla Foundation, we take on this mission with a strategic focus and an unshakeable resolve. Together with our partners, we move forward with hope, determined to make palliative care possible for those who need it the most.'

One of the best examples of integration after Kalwa Hospital is that under the Brihanmumbai Municipal Corporation (BMC), all four of the medical colleges now have either paediatric or adult palliative care services available. The first was Nair Municipal Hospital in 2021 for paediatrics, then in subsequent years King Edward Memorial Hospital for neonatal palliative care and Sion for paediatrics. Dr Rustom Narsi Cooper Municipal General Hospital has just started adult palliative care services.

Dr Mohan Joshi, dean at Sion Hospital, Mumbai, says, 'The introduction of palliative care across neonatology, paediatrics and adult services at Sion has been transformative. It is proving that even in a busy tertiary-level municipal hospital, excellence in service and patient-centred care is achievable. By listening more closely to patients with serious illnesses, providing them with the information they need and maintaining follow-ups post discharge, we are extending holistic care that truly makes a difference.'

For families, this means less stress and fewer financial burdens. For hospitals, it eases the load on doctors and improves overall care. Including palliative care in healthcare makes the approach more humane and thoughtful. For, no one should feel alone when facing one of life's hardest journeys.

Dr Sangeeta Ravat, dean at King Edward Memorial Hospital, the first BMC hospital to start neonatal palliative care in the city, agrees: 'We have witnessed the profound impact of palliative care on easing the suffering of our most vulnerable patients. When a mother learns that her baby has a chronic, lifelong condition or faces a shorter life, the palliative care team steps in to provide compassionate support.

From running support groups to offering follow-up care for families, together with the best medical treatment for the child, we are demonstrating that a continuum of care is possible even in a bustling government hospital.'

Palliative Care in the Private Sector

In my meeting with Dr Sujeet Rajan, Bhatia Hospital, he says: 'As the private sector plays an important role for healthcare in India, it is important that these hospital administrators and health professionals also appreciate the value that palliative care adds to the overall journey of a patient and their satisfaction with hospital services.'

'I see hospitals claim that they have complete cancer care. How can they call themselves complete if they do not have a palliative care department?' asks Dr Sultan Pradhan, of Punyashlok Ahilyadevi Holkar Head and Neck Cancer Institute of India, Mumbai. While he believes that every doctor should wear a 'palliative care lens' all the time, he did set up a separate palliative and supportive care OPD within the hospital to address the needs of patients with complex pain and symptoms, those requiring more information about the disease, having challenging family situations or struggling with resources.

The Institute has been in operation for a year at the time of writing. 'Looking back at the last year,' Dr Pradhan says, 'this team has been a tremendous support to the oncologists here, following up with patients who may have dropped out of treatment and supporting emotionally not only the patient but also the caregivers.'

As palliative care gets embedded in both public and private sectors, there needs to be greater awareness about the value of palliative care as well as the need for more healthcare professionals to train in palliative medicine. Only then can the vision of compassionate and holistic care become a reality for everyone who needs it.

10

A Good Life

'You matter because you are you. You matter to the last moment of your life, and we will do all we can not only to help you die peacefully but to live until you die.'

– DR CICELY SAUNDERS

So, when should palliative care begin? Ideally, right at the start, with the diagnosis. CanSupport's Harmala Gupta says: 'Someone who has received a diagnosis that is life-altering like cancer needs psychosocial support from day one. They need psychological support to understand what they are going through. They need social support, they need to be educated about the illness, and the caregivers need to know about how they will have to care for this person now. We have to have open discussions about these things and the fact that we must also educate the larger community so that people don't think it's a disease that you can spread by touching someone because we often found, when we went into homes, that patients were isolated, grandchildren weren't allowed to meet them because the parents would say, "No-no-no, you'll get the disease," and sometimes even the patients would believe this. Their clothes were washed separately, their dishes were washed separately because we have had a history of communicable diseases, and this is what is applied to the world of cancer as well.'

The standard model suggests that at the start of the disease, there is a small component of palliative care and a large component of medical care. As the disease progresses, the role of palliative care increases as the curative component decreases, until the patient arrives at the end-of-life stage where palliative care takes over symptom management, pain relief and the psychological aspects of preparing the patient and the family for death.

In a busy hospital, doctors may see so many patients a day that it is evident that even if a small percentage of them receive these diagnoses, the doctors will not have the time to deal with anything more than diagnosis and prescription. Thus, current wisdom suggests that palliative care should work side by side with the medical team.

Timing is everything. Again and again, palliative care specialists say that it is wrong to begin palliative care only when the doctor can 'no longer do anything'.

Dr C.S. Pramesh, director, TMH, Mumbai, says: 'Associating palliative care with end-of-life care is a misnomer because palliative care includes symptom control and this is important even in the earlier stages of the disease. Early involvement helps patients feel seen and heard, reduces feelings of abandonment and ensures that their emotional physical and spiritual needs are met every step of the way. When curative care and palliative care work together seamlessly, it creates a smoother experience for everyone, making difficult decisions easier and providing continuous support for both the patient and their loved ones.'

This seamlessness is part of giving patients the care and comfort they deserve at every level. It helps preserve the dignity of each human life. When one looks around a public hospital, this may seem impossible. There is just so much suffering, there are so many sick people, so little by way of resources. The resource crunch is not just one that public hospitals face.

'Consider a good death,' says Smriti Rana, head, Strategic Programs and Partnerships, Pallium India. 'Historically, a good end has been defined as dying at home, without pain, with your issues resolved and your loved ones all around you. But is that what a good death looks like in India? In this country, it could well just be a death without pain, a death without fighting for the next breath, irrespective of where you die. So even the idea of a good death has been whitewashed. Yes, it should be with your loved ones around you, but if your home is under a flyover, would you want to die there? You might want to die in a hospice under professional palliative care.'

Sadly, even when you have the resources, you may die in an ICU, which most doctors would admit is not the best place to bid farewell.

Dr Minnie Bodhanwala, CEO, Wadia Hospitals, Mumbai, says, 'I've witnessed first hand how healthcare expenditure in chronic illness often disproportionately increases in the final months of a patient's life. There is a significant push for hospitalization, invasive procedures and treatments in an attempt to save the patient at any cost, even when the likelihood of success is minimal. While well intentioned, these interventions frequently lead to mounting medical bills that contribute little to improving the quality of life for the patient. The very nature of these interventions can reduce the patient's quality of life in their final months. The long-term financial and emotional consequences of medical costs on families, especially those who are forced into bankruptcy and intergenerational debt, are truly heart-wrenching. Palliative care is a true game changer for both families and patients. When introduced early, palliative care shifts the focus from aggressive, often ineffective treatments to a more holistic approach.'

Smriti Rana adds, 'I don't know if you know this but in 2014 and in 2020, the National Crime Record Bureau revealed that the second highest reason for suicide is living with an illness. The highest is "domestic issues"; the second highest, nearly 20 per cent is "a chronic advanced illness". Now there is no study that tells you why this is the case, but if you apply your mind, you can tell. Either they're a financial burden on the family or their pain is uncontrolled, their suffering unaddressed. Every year, 55 million Indians are pushed below the poverty line because of out-of-pocket catastrophic healthcare expenditure. I would rather end my life than bring multigenerational debt on my family. Although a straight line hasn't been drawn between these statistics, it's not rocket science.'

While the ICU at times is the only option for patients and families, dying in an ICU can also mean dying alone since families cannot see their patients freely. And so, it has been agreed generally that the best place to die is the family home. But this may not always be possible for a number of reasons – lack of space, absence of a carer, distress and pain that requires medical attention or the inability of the family to witness such distress. In that case, a palliative care centre or a hospice may be a better space to die than in an ICU. But it is not an easy decision to make, not in India.

'Social pressure – the real or imagined opinion of others – plays a huge role in Indian life,' says Dr Sushma Bhatnagar, clinical lead and senior consultant, Pain, Palliative Medicine and Supportive Care, Indraprastha Apollo Hospitals. 'Many people view ICU care as "doing everything possible" because it's often associated with aggressive treatments and the hope of saving a life. On the other hand, palliative care is sometimes wrongly seen as "giving up", because it focusses on comfort rather than trying to cure the illness. Cultural beliefs can play a big role in these decisions – some cultures emphasize fighting for life at all costs. It's important to understand that accepting the natural progression of life and preparing for a good death doesn't mean giving up. Ultimately, it's about focusing on a life well lived, and when the time comes, helping people transition with peace, surrounded by love and care.'

The medical profession has also been trained to see death as failure. Dr Anupama Borkar, Goa Medical College, says, 'Doctors see it as their moral responsibility to fight for the patient until the last breath. It's not easy, but that mindset has to change. The death of a patient is not a failure. Death is inevitable; it is what happens to all those who have been given the gift of life. We must train the younger generation to accept this, and to help our patients die a good death, in peace, made as comfortable as possible and with their loved ones around them.'

The Business of Preventing Regrets

Death and taxes, Benjamin Franklin told us, are inevitable. Often it seems that more planning goes into taxes than into death. And really, planning does help a great deal. It even helps deal with fear.

At the International Conference of the IAPC in 2024, I remember Dr Justin Baker putting it beautifully:

'We have to be in the regret-preventing business.' And if you don't acknowledge the fact that someone you love is going to die, you can't plan for it, you can't help them plan for it, you can't help them finish up unfinished business, and that can only lead to regrets.

Mary, a patient with stage 4 oral cancer at Karunashraya, knew that her end was coming. The family had dispensed with collusion and had told her. She said that she had always been a good cook and would like to leave her recipes behind. And so, the homecare team found someone to help her put her recipes down and they printed copies of the cookbook.

I am the proud owner of one copy of the limited edition of Mary's book of recipes.

In the future, we will have a medical system that will be truly patient-centred, but right now it is better to have the difficult conversations about whether you want to be resuscitated or not, about whether you want to be put on a ventilator or not when you are still in good health. Clear directives will help make sure your wishes are respected for doctors are often confused when families agree on one thing in the evening and after a conference call with a sibling or a child in some other part of the world, reverse the decision in the morning.

Embracing Grief, Honouring Life

Harsh was eleven years old when he died. 'It is surprising how many children want to go home in the last stages. They want to make one last visit to their native place,' says Ramalakshmi, palliative care coordinator at Golden Butterflies in Chennai. 'We encourage the parents to make this possible. We prepare them for all the things that they need to know. We make contact with local doctors and explain the situation.'

Perhaps it is a return to a place where they were happy when school was out and report cards far away, where grandparents would welcome them and there would be dips in the local river, fruit from the trees and late nights under the stars.

We arrive and find Harsh's mother and her sister waiting for us. Ramalakshmi takes their hands. They begin to cry and tell her about his last days. He was a creative child who liked working with lights. Harsh illuminated photo frames for the family and for the neighbours. There is a picture of him in one of the small rooms, and it is garlanded with a set of fairy lights.

Harsh has a younger brother, Parth, a preschooler, who hangs around, looking at all of us with the big, curious eyes of a child. But when anyone approaches, Parth shrinks away, into himself. Suddenly, he starts to cry, and his mother picks him up and cuddles him. He goes limp, his cheek pressed into her shoulder.

If this has been a stressful time for the entire family, Parth has also had it tough. Until recently, he had an elder brother. It is likely that he loved his elder brother but also resented the attention he got from everyone in equal measure. It is also likely that he feels guilty about Harsh's death in a manner that he has no way of articulating.

Harsh was not told that he was dying. This is not uncommon. Parents do not think children will understand the 'D word' but since they were willing to talk to the palliative care team, they could plan a little and they could grant their son his wish to go back to the village.

Harsh's mother tells us that this is the first day that the house will be empty of all the relatives who have visited. She will now have to get used to the empty space in the room. Her sister, who has been standing behind her through all this like a rock, says that they watched over his sleep until about two in the morning and then dozed off. When they woke up, around six, he was gone.

It seems a common phenomenon among children, waiting until they are alone. One has heard of children sending their parents' home to sleep and then slipping off to keep their appointment with death. We want so much to believe that we are strong and the loved one is weak. But the person in pain has grown in strength, has matured beyond their age.

The bereavement visit here takes nearly an hour. There is no attempt to console, no attempt to explain. It is a moment to share. All the mental health professionals I met emphasized that grief was a natural response to bereavement.

Dr Ira Almeida's team in South Goa watches for what is known as complicated grief, where the intensity of the pain does not seem to ebb and one cannot get back to the ordinary routines of life. 'Fifteen days after the death, we do a physical visit. On the third monthly visit, we screen the family for complicated grief. Yes, grief after bereavement is natural, but eventually one has to get back to work and get back to the normal routine. If you can't, it means you have complicated grief. On the first of every month, we call up everyone, but if there is a case of complicated grief the team must go in person.'

Loss is never easy. But even a difficult situation can be eased somewhat by grief and bereavement counselling. Grief has its own internal timetable, its own logic. Weeping taps into grief and, we are told, externalizes it, helps us to deal with the peculiar insistent pressure that builds up as the world sails calmly on the outside.

As the Marathi bhakti poet Muktabai wrote seven centuries ago:

First came joy and on the morrow
Hard on her heels, a visit from sorrow
Just as well settled down to grieving
She announced that she was leaving ... [6]

As I crossed the country to watch palliative care in action, I began to feel a change come over me.

In the writing of this book, I have seen how much our shared humanity achieves in compassion and empathy. I have seen how pain is part of the human condition, but equally how much there is of love and courage and hope.

The palliative care approach for me is an acceptance that the one thing we can all be sure of – if we win the Great Lottery of Birth – it is that we must some day die. To live fully, in comfort and with dignity to our last day is the greatest affirmation of life. To make this possible has to be the biggest gift we can give others and ourselves.

Pain Is Inevitable, Suffering Is Not

This is the central message of all the stories in the pages of this book – stories of those who care, those who need care, those who have the courage to accept that they need care and those who have the empathy and compassion to provide it.

Through my journey, I have experienced the power of stories, the wonder of making a human connection.

Listening to other people, letting ourselves into their life experience when they open the door for us, will make us less ignorant, less fearful; it can open us up to the possibility of compassion for others as much as for ourselves. Many people have shared their lives courageously with me. Such wisdom as there is between the covers of this book has been lent to me; the mistakes are mine.

The last eighteen months of researching and writing this book have given me some sense of the inner resources of the human being; that one can face whatever life throws at one, as long as one is willing to accept help and as long as that help is offered on an egalitarian basis. I cannot say I am no longer afraid of pain. But I think I can say that it seems now that the moment calls up the resources, the need brings forth what is needed. Of this, we build our faith in the future.

Welcome to the gentle revolution of palliative medicine, the gentle revolution of caring.

Notes

1. Tata Memorial Hospital (TMH) in Mumbai was the first hospital in what has now grown into a nationwide network. It currently operates under the Tata Memorial Centre (TMC), which oversees TMH along with a growing network of affiliated cancer care and research institutions across India.
2. 'Palliative Care', World Health Organization, 5 August 2020, https://www.who.int/news-room/fact-sheets/detail/palliative-care.
3. 'Palliative Care Is Integral to a Caring Health System', Civil Society, 29 July 2023, https://www.civilsocietyonline.com/interviews/palliative-care-is-integral-to-a-caring-health-system/.
4. CBS Handbook on Pain & Palliative Care, Sarita Singh and Manish Kumar Singh, CBS Publishers and Distributors Pvt. Ltd, 2023.
5. https://my.clevelandclinic.org/health/diseases/9225-caregiver-burnout; accessed on 25 March 2024.
6. From *The Ant Who Swallowed the Sun: The Abhangs of the Marathi Women Saints*, translated by Neela Bhagwat and Jerry Pinto (Speaking Tiger, 2019).

How Can I Find Palliative Care?

SAATH-SAATH HELPLINE
1800-202-7777
Open Monday to Saturday, 10 a.m. to 6 p.m.

The Saath-Saath helpline is a collaborative effort of palliative care organizations across India with a shared vision to support people with any serious illness, their caregivers and healthcare professionals.

This national toll-free number is staffed by trained palliative care volunteers who listen, assess the callers' need and link them to the nearest palliative care provider. Saath-Saath could make all the difference to someone who might be in pain, is alone and needs support, by connecting them to a world of information and compassion.

Acknowledgments

I'm deeply grateful to everyone who trusted me with their experiences and helped bring this book to life.

This is as much your story as it is mine.

To the doctors, palliative care professionals, patients and their families: thank you for sharing your time and wisdom with such honesty and heart. Your endurance, empathy and grace have left me with lessons I'll carry forever.

To Ravi Singh, friend, philosopher, guide, many thanks for being the sounding board for this book. I have had a career in publishing because of you.

And to everyone at the Veha Foundation who were instrumental in getting this book off the ground, into the air and into your hands.